# The Vagus Lifestyle

Daily Habits and Simple Practices to Live Longer, Sleep

Better, and Strengthen Your Body's Natural Healing Power

Nicci Brochard
&
Dr. Ben Chuba

# The Vagus Lifestyle

Daily Habits and Simple Practices to Live Longer, Sleep
Better, and Strengthen Your Body's Natural Healing Power

Book Formatting by: Monisha

Book cover design by: *Billy Design*

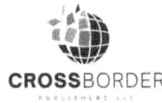

**CROSS**BORDER

New York, London, Quebec

# Contents

## Chapter 6: Gut Feelings – Nutrition, Digestion, and the Vagus Nerve ...................................................................................... 87

## Chapter 7: The Vagus Lifestyle in Action – Your Daily Plan for Long-Term Wellness..............................................................103

## Epilogue..............................................................................126

# Introduction

Deep within your body runs a superhighway of healing that most people never learn to access. The vagus nerve—your longest cranial nerve—extends from your brainstem down through your neck, chest, and abdomen, connecting your brain to your heart, lungs, digestive system, and beyond. This remarkable neural pathway holds the key to transforming your health, yet modern medicine has only recently begun to understand its profound influence on longevity, sleep quality, immune function, and emotional well-being.

Ancient wisdom traditions have long recognized the power of breath, meditation, and mindful living to promote healing. Now, cutting-edge neuroscience reveals that these practices specifically activate your vagus nerve, triggering your body's natural relaxation response and unleashing its innate capacity for repair and regeneration.

Every day, millions of people struggle with chronic stress, poor sleep, digestive issues, and inflammatory conditions—all signs of an underactive vagus nerve. The pharmaceutical industry offers temporary fixes, but the real solution lies in reawakening this built-in healing system through simple, scientifically-backed lifestyle modifications.

The practices you'll discover in these pages require no special equipment, expensive supplements, or dramatic life overhauls. Cold exposure, specific breathing techniques, gentle movement, mindful eating, and strategic social connections can dramatically improve your vagal tone within weeks. These aren't complex medical interventions— they're accessible daily habits that our ancestors practiced instinctively.

Your vagus nerve responds to consistency rather than intensity. Small, purposeful actions repeated daily create profound shifts in how your nervous system functions. The transformation begins the moment you understand that your body already possesses everything needed for optimal health.

The journey toward vibrant longevity starts with a single conscious breath. Your healing superhighway awaits activation, and the tools for unlocking its power rest entirely within your hands.

Ben and I (Nicci) thank you immensely for choosing our book. We promise you a great time ahead.

# Chapter 1

# Meet Your Vagus Nerve – The Body's Secret to Self-Healing

## A Real-Life Healing Journey

Every healing journey begins with a story. Meet Leah, a 45-year-old professional who found herself at a breaking point. Years of high-pressure work and personal turmoil had pushed Leah into a state of chronic stress. She was suffering from relentless anxiety, barely sleeping three hours a night, and plagued by stress-related health issues – frequent tension headaches, a nervous stomach that left her nauseous at mealtimes, and heart palpitations that sent her into panic. When traditional medicine offered little more than pills for anxiety and insomnia, Leah felt stuck in a cycle of symptom management rather than true healing.

Desperate for relief, Leah stumbled upon a local wellness class that taught deep breathing and meditation. With nothing to lose, she decided to give it a try. On her first evening in class, as she sat on the yoga mat learning to slow down her breath, Leah experienced something remarkable. After about ten minutes of diaphragmatic breathing – inhaling deeply into her belly and exhaling slowly – she felt an unfamiliar calm wash over her. Her racing heart gradually steadied. The tightness in her chest eased. For the first time in months, she left the class with her mind quiet and her body at ease. That night, Leah slept a full seven hours. It was as if she had flipped a switch inside her body that shifted it from chaos to calm.

Encouraged by this progress, Leah made these breathing exercises and a short mindfulness meditation part of her daily routine. Each morning, she spent 15 minutes practicing slow, rhythmic breathing and gentle meditation. Over the weeks, her symptoms started to fade. The headaches became rare. Her digestion improved and the queasy, nervous stomach settled down. She had more energy during the day and noticed her mood lifting. Friends remarked that she seemed "more like herself" again – calm, resilient, and even glowing. Leah herself was astonished; these simple mind-body practices were succeeding where medications had failed.

Curious to understand why breathing and meditation were so transformative, Leah dug into the science and learned about a powerful nerve running through her body – something called the vagus nerve. It turned out that every time she engaged in slow breathing or entered a meditative state, she was activating her vagus nerve, sending signals of safety and relaxation throughout her system. This in turn was triggering her body's self-healing processes – lowering her stress hormones, reducing inflammation, and allowing her mind and body to rebalance. The more consistently she practiced, the stronger this calming pathway became. In essence, Leah had tapped into her body's *secret self-healing switch*, and it was the vagus nerve all along.

Leah's story is real (with her name changed for privacy) and illustrative. It shows how tapping into the vagus nerve's power can lead to profound improvements in health. A woman on the brink of collapse from chronic stress recovered her vitality through practices that anyone can do – no fancy equipment or prescriptions needed. This compelling journey sets the stage for our exploration of the vagus nerve. How can one nerve wield so much influence over our well-being? And more importantly, how can *you* harness it to live healthier and happier? Let's begin by getting to know this nerve that quietly connects and balances nearly every major system in your body.

## The Body's Control Center – Vagus Nerve 101

Hidden within your body's nervous system is a multitasking marvel called the vagus nerve. If you've never heard of it, you're not alone – for years it's been the body's best-kept secret. Often nicknamed the "information superhighway" between brain and body, the vagus nerve is the longest of all your cranial nerves. It originates at the base of your brain (in the brainstem) and wanders through your body (in fact, *vagus* comes from the Latin word for "wandering"). True to its name, it travels from your brain down your neck and into your chest and abdomen, branching out like a tree to touch almost every major organ along the way. It connects to your heart, lungs, stomach, intestines, liver, kidneys, and even your voice box. Think of the vagus nerve as a communication cable linking your brain to your vital organs – constantly sending signals back and forth to keep your body in balance.

What does this "superhighway" carry? Crucial information. The vagus nerve helps control a wide range of automatic processes that keep you alive and well. For example, it relays signals that regulate your heart rate and blood pressure. A healthy vagus nerve gently slows the heart down after a scare or exertion, preventing it from beating too fast for too long. It also influences your breathing and respiratory rate, telling your lungs when to relax and breathe deeply. Digestion, too, is under vagal control – when you eat, it's the vagus nerve that nudges your stomach to produce digestive juices and move food along your intestines. Ever notice your stomach "knot" when you're anxious? That's vagus-driven communication in action, illustrating how our gut and brain are linked by this very nerve. The vagus also plays a role in managing mood and emotional well-being: it connects to areas of the brain that regulate anxiety and happiness, and it helps release neurotransmitters like acetylcholine and serotonin which can uplift mood and sharpen memory. Even your immune system and inflammation response are influenced by the vagus nerve – it can signal the body to tone down inflammation when it's no longer needed, acting as an internal anti-inflammatory circuit. This is why Cedars-Sinai medical experts refer to the vagus nerve as an internal "brake" on the inflammatory response – an essential function, since runaway inflammation is at the root of many diseases.

Crucially, the vagus nerve is the captain of your parasympathetic nervous system, often known as the "rest and digest" system. You might recall from basic biology that the autonomic nervous system has two major divisions: the sympathetic ("fight or flight") and the parasympathetic ("rest and digest"). These two work in tandem, like a seesaw, to keep you balanced. When you're confronted with danger or stress, the sympathetic side kicks in to pump you up – heart rate surges, breathing quickens, muscles tense, and stress hormones flood your bloodstream. That reaction helps you spring into action or stay alert. But you're not meant to live in fight-or-flight mode forever; this is where the parasympathetic system comes in. Once the danger passes, the vagus nerve jumps into action to counteract stress and trigger relaxation. It's essentially your body's natural reset button. The vagus nerve sends out calming signals: your heart rate slows back down, blood pressure drops to normal, breathing becomes deeper and slower, and digestion resumes. You might even feel a yawn or a deep exhale – classic signs that the vagus-induced relaxation response is taking over. In this restful state, your body can focus on maintenance and healing: digesting food, repairing cells, and restoring equilibrium.

To appreciate the vagus nerve's importance, imagine it as a command center for healing. When activated, it shifts multiple organs and systems into a "healing mode." Your heart relaxes, your gut works efficiently, and even your immune cells get the message to reduce unnecessary inflammation. It's as if the vagus nerve orchestrates a symphony where each instrument is a body part, all playing a calm, harmonious tune. This is why stimulating the vagus nerve can feel like a wave of calm washing over you – it physiologically *turns on* calmness and recovery. In Leah's story above, those deep breaths she took weren't just "in her head" relaxing her; they were literally activating vagus nerve fibers in her diaphragm and chest, which signaled her brain to shift into parasympathetic gear. The result was a cascade of physical changes –

slower heartbeat, muscle relaxation, quieter thoughts – that helped her body start to heal.

Science is only beginning to fully map the influence of this nerve, but what we know so far is incredible. The vagus nerve has a hand in regulating mood, digestion, heart function, respiratory rate, inflammatory responses, and more – all at the same time! Because of this broad reach, some scientists call the vagus nerve a "mind-body nexus": it's a tangible, biological link between our mental state and physical health. When something goes wrong with vagal signaling, the effects can show up just about anywhere in the body. Conversely, when we find ways to improve vagus nerve function (as Leah did, unknowingly at first), we can positively influence many aspects of our health at once.

So, in "Vagus Nerve 101," the key takeaway is this: your vagus nerve is the master communicator and calming force in your body. It constantly works to rebalance you after stress, keep your vital organs functioning optimally, and even helps rein in damaging inflammation. It's the built-in mechanism that makes self-healing possible, by promoting what doctors sometimes refer to as the "relaxation response" – a state in which your body can restore and repair itself. Understanding this remarkable nerve sets the stage for everything else in this book. With the basics under our belt, let's explore why having a *strong* vagus nerve (something we call high *vagal tone*) matters so much for long-term health and vitality.

## Vagal Tone and Vitality – Why It Matters

By now you can sense that the vagus nerve is vital for day-to-day balance, but the story doesn't end with short-term relaxation. The strength or activity level of your vagus nerve – known as vagal tone – has profound implications for your long-term health. *Vagal tone* essentially refers to how effective the vagus nerve is at doing its job. You can think of it like muscle tone: a well-trained muscle responds quickly and efficiently when you need it. Similarly, a "toned" vagus nerve responds readily to keep you calm, regulate your organs, and buffer stress. High vagal tone means your body can easily activate the vagus nerve's calming, healing influence; low vagal tone means that signal is weaker and slower, so it's harder for you to come down from stress arousal.

Why does vagal tone matter? Research over the past two decades has unveiled that people with higher vagal tone tend to be healthier, more resilient, and even live longer than those with low vagal tone. This makes sense, because high vagal tone is associated with a well-balanced autonomic nervous system – your "rest and digest" response can kick in appropriately to counteract stress. For example, individuals with high vagal tone often have a lower resting heart rate and higher heart rate variability (HRV), which is a measure of the healthy fluctuations in time between heartbeats. Higher HRV (a hallmark of good vagal tone) correlates with lower risk of cardiac events and better cardiovascular fitness. High vagal tone also links to better digestion and less trouble with gut disorders like irritable bowel syndrome. In terms of mental health, numerous studies have found that people with robust vagal activity handle stress better and are less prone to severe anxiety or depression – essentially, their nervous system is more adept at bouncing back from challenges. Even sleep quality appears to improve with higher vagal tone; a balanced nervous system promotes deeper, more restorative sleep, whereas an overactive stress response can lead to insomnia or restless nights.

One of the most important benefits of a strong vagus nerve is its role in controlling inflammation. Chronic inflammation is a driving factor in aging and in diseases ranging from arthritis and heart disease to diabetes and dementia. Remarkably, the vagus nerve helps keep this in check through what scientists call the "inflammatory reflex." When the vagus nerve is stimulated, it sends signals that *reduce the production of pro-inflammatory molecules* in the body. In other words, a high vagal tone can put the brakes on runaway inflammation, preventing your immune system from overreacting and damaging healthy tissue. This keeps your immune system in balance – ready to fight invaders when necessary, but not perpetually on high alert. Think of inflammation like a small fire that's useful for clearing debris or fighting infection in the body; the vagus nerve ensures that once the job is done, the fire is damped down so it doesn't spread and burn everything. People with higher vagal tone generally have lower levels of inflammatory markers in their bloodstream. This is a big reason why high vagal tone is linked to *healthier aging*. By keeping chronic inflammation at bay, the vagus nerve helps protect you from the "slow burn" damage that accumulates over years and contributes to aging and organ deterioration.

The scientific evidence for vagal tone's impact on vitality is truly exciting. In fact, a groundbreaking study in the U.K. provided a dramatic example of what boosting vagal tone might achieve. Researchers at the University of Leeds conducted an experiment with adults over age 55, using a gentle form of daily vagus nerve stimulation. The method was intriguingly simple: participants "tickled" their vagus nerve using a mild electrical current applied to a spot on the outer ear (the ear happens to have a branch of the vagus nerve accessible at the surface). They did this for just 15 minutes a day over two weeks. The results were eye-opening. After this short period, the seniors showed a measurable increase in vagal tone – their parasympathetic activity went up and the overactive sympathetic "fight or flight" activity went down, rebalancing their autonomic nervous system. Many participants reported improvements in mood and significant enhancements in sleep quality. Some who had been waking frequently at night or feeling low and anxious found themselves sleeping more soundly and experiencing brighter, more stable moods during the day. Essentially, by *gently stimulating their vagus nerve*, they were able to reverse some effects of stress and aging in just days.

The researchers were enthusiastic about what this could mean for healthy aging. When the body's stress and relaxation systems were rebalanced, the participants' overall risk factors for chronic illness seemed to improve. In fact, maintaining a healthier autonomic balance (more "rest and digest," less chronic "fight or flight") is associated with lower risk of age-related diseases like high blood pressure and heart disease. Moreover, it can even correspond with a lower risk of mortality – yes, a lower risk of death – in older adults. By the study's end, those with the initially weakest vagal tone (the most imbalanced nervous systems) showed the greatest improvements, suggesting that boosting vagal tone could be most life-changing for those who need it most. One of the lead scientists, Dr. Beatrice Bretherton, noted that using the ear's vagus nerve branch was like opening a "gateway" to the body's internal control system, potentially slowing down some processes of aging without any drugs or invasive procedures. She went on to say the impressive results they saw were likely "just the tip of the iceberg" – hinting that longer-term or earlier interventions could yield even more substantial health benefits. Another senior researcher, Dr. Susan Deuchars, remarked that this simple daily therapy had the potential to *make a big difference in people's lives* and could eventually be applied to help various disorders of aging.

What all this research means for us is powerful: nurturing your vagus nerve isn't just about feeling relaxed in the moment – it could influence how well you age and how strong your body remains over the years. High vagal tone has been correlated with what some call "successful aging," marked by preserved cognitive function, robust emotional health, and resistance to disease. Conversely, low vagal tone has been observed in many chronic conditions – for example, people with depression, PTSD, or chronic inflammatory diseases often exhibit lower vagal activity. This doesn't mean low vagal tone caused those issues, but it does suggest that improving vagal tone might help protect against or mitigate such conditions.

To sum it up, vagal tone is a vital sign of vitality. When you take steps to strengthen your vagus nerve (and we will soon talk about how to do that), you are potentially stacking the odds in favor of a longer and healthier life. You're helping your body keep inflammation in check, maintain equilibrium under stress, sleep deeply, and recover faster. It's like giving yourself an insurance policy against the wear and tear of life. The evidence we have – from correlations with longevity to direct studies like the "ear tickle therapy" – all builds the case that caring for your vagus nerve is an investment in your future self. Just as exercising your muscles can keep you physically fit, exercising your vagus nerve can keep your entire mind-body system resilient.

Think of a high vagal tone as a state of thriving: your heart is steady and strong, your digestion is smooth, your mind is centered, and your immune system is vigilant but cool-headed. In this state, you wake up feeling refreshed, you handle challenges with more ease, and your body bounces back quickly whether you've had a stressful day or you're fighting off a cold. That's the vitality we're talking about. And the wonderful news is that vagal tone isn't fixed – you can improve it with simple practices. The rest of this book is devoted to showing you how. But before we dive into the specific habits and exercises, let's look at the big picture of what adopting a "vagus lifestyle" means, and how these small daily changes can yield *outsized* benefits for your health and well-being.

## The Vagus Lifestyle Overview

By now, you might be thinking, "This sounds amazing – but how do I actually *strengthen* my vagus nerve?" That question lies at the heart of this book. "The vagus lifestyle" is the term we'll use to describe a new approach to daily living that prioritizes and improves vagal tone. It's about integrating simple, science-backed habits into your routine that consistently engage your vagus nerve's healing powers. The beauty of the vagus lifestyle is that it doesn't require drastic changes or expensive interventions. In fact, many of the most effective vagus-friendly practices are deceptively simple – things you can do at home, at no cost, for just a few minutes a day. Yet their impact can transform how you feel on a daily basis.

So what kinds of habits are we talking about? Here's a sneak peek of what's to come in the chapters ahead, where we blend cutting-edge science with practical techniques:

- **Deep Breathing Exercises:** Remember how Leah's first big breakthrough came from breathing? We'll explore specific breathing techniques – from diaphragmatic breathing to patterns like 4-7-8 breathing – that directly stimulate the vagus nerve and bring about calm. Just a few minutes of slow, deep belly breathing sends a signal up the vagus nerve that it's "time to relax," slowing your heart and triggering a relaxation response throughout the body. This can be done anytime, anywhere to quickly dial down stress and even help you fall asleep more easily.

- **Mindfulness and Meditation:** These practices train your nervous system to stay in the present and activate your parasympathetic "rest and digest" mode. We'll cover beginner-friendly mindfulness exercises and meditation techniques (no prior experience needed) that have been shown to boost vagal tone. For example, research shows that even brief daily meditation can increase vagus activity and lead to improvements in mood and attention. You'll learn how focusing your mind and breathing can become a powerful vagus nerve workout that also clears mental clutter and anxiety.

- **Cold Exposure (Therapeutic Cold):** It might sound intimidating, but simple forms of cold exposure – like a 30-second cool rinse at the end of your shower or dunking your face in cold water – can strongly activate the vagus nerve. Athletes and wellness enthusiasts have popularized cold showers and ice baths for their invigorating benefits. We'll demystify the science behind this: cold stimulation prompts a reflex that increases vagus nerve signals, which in turn can slow heart rate and reduce inflammation. You'll discover safe, gentle ways to use cold as a tool to reset your nervous system (no polar bear plunge required, unless you're up for it!).

- **Diet Tweaks for Vagal Tone:** Food isn't just fuel; it's information for your nervous system and gut, which is tightly linked to the vagus nerve. We'll discuss how certain dietary choices can support vagus nerve function – for instance, foods rich in omega-3 fatty acids (found in fish and flaxseeds) are known to support nerve health and have anti-inflammatory properties that complement vagus activity. A diet high in natural fiber from fruits and vegetables supports a healthy gut microbiome, which communicates with the brain via the vagus nerve (often called the gut-brain axis). We'll also cover mindful eating practices – like eating slowly and chewing thoroughly – which engage the vagus nerve to enhance digestion and satiety signals. These are small tweaks that can make your meals into vagus-friendly rituals.

- **Joyful Movement and Exercise:** Gentle exercise, especially activities like yoga, tai chi, or even a relaxed walk in nature, can stimulate vagal tone. Unlike high-intensity workouts that rev up your sympathetic system, these mindful movements balance exertion with relaxation. Yoga, in particular, has been shown to increase heart rate variability (a sign of vagus activation) and improve mood. We'll highlight how incorporating regular physical activity that you *enjoy* – whether it's dancing, cycling, or gardening – contributes to a healthier nervous system. Exercise also helps you sleep better and reduces baseline stress, indirectly supporting vagal tone.

- **Social Connection and Laughter:** Believe it or not, spending time with loved ones or even playing with a pet can activate your vagus nerve. Positive social interactions – talking, laughing, hugging – release oxytocin and create a sense of safety, which stimulates the vagus-driven relaxation response. We'll talk about the importance of community, laughter, and even singing (yes, singing aloud or humming stimulates the vocal cords and vagus nerve) as part of the vagus lifestyle. A simple habit like calling a friend or having a hearty laugh each day is not just good for the soul, it's good for your vagus nerve too!

Throughout the upcoming chapters, each of these habits (and more) will be unpacked in detail. You'll learn why they work – the science of how they affect your body – and how to do them step by step. What's truly empowering is understanding that these practices trigger real, physiological changes. For instance, when you take those slow breaths or finish a cold shower and feel refreshed, it's not just in your head – it's your vagus nerve shifting your body into a state of balance and repair. Bit by bit, day by day, these habits build your vagal tone, much like regular exercise builds muscle. And as your vagal tone grows, you'll likely notice you feel calmer, sleep more deeply, digest better, and have more emotional resilience in the face of life's ups and downs.

The vagus lifestyle is a new paradigm in wellness because it leverages *small daily actions for disproportionately large gains*. In a world that often suggests that "more is better" – more intense workouts, stricter diets, or heavy-duty interventions – the vagus lifestyle offers a refreshing alternative. It's about working *with* your body's natural healing systems rather than against them. Think of it as learning to play your body's built-in instrument (the vagus nerve) to produce harmony from within. Instead of just addressing surface symptoms, you'll be tuning the "conductor" that directs many systems at once. This holistic, inside-out approach can lead to improvements that sometimes surprise even medical professionals. It's not unusual, for example, for someone practicing vagus-friendly habits to report that their blood pressure normalized, their chronic pain lessened, or that they finally shed those few extra pounds – not because those were directly targeted, but because the body as a whole moved into a state of better balance and healing.

Ultimately, the goal of the vagus lifestyle is to empower you. You'll come to understand that you hold a powerful key to your well-being – the ability to consciously influence your vagus nerve. This understanding alone is uplifting: it shifts you from a passive role (where health is something that happens *to* you) to an active role (where health is something you actively cultivate). As physicians at Massachusetts General Hospital have noted in their patient guidance, simply knowing about the vagus nerve and how to engage it can help you take *proactive steps to improve your health and quality of life*. It's like being handed the user manual to a complex machine you've been operating your whole life without instructions – suddenly, things make a lot more sense, and you can optimize the settings.

In the chapters ahead, as we dive into each habit and practice, keep Leah's story in mind – and know that her outcome is very much achievable for you. You do not need to be at a crisis point to benefit; whether you're health-conscious and looking to optimize wellness, dealing with a chronic illness, or a wellness professional seeking new tools for clients, the vagus lifestyle offers something valuable. It meets you where you are and helps you get to a better place. If you're struggling with stress, you'll learn ways to find calm each day. If you're aiming for longevity, you'll discover techniques that could help you live not just longer but better. And if you're on a healing journey from any condition, these practices will become allies in your recovery, strengthening your body's natural healing power.

As we wrap up this introductory chapter, imagine the possibilities. Picture being able to fall asleep peacefully at night because you have a go-to breathing exercise that quiets your mind. Envision tackling your day with a resilient mood, because your morning meditation has strengthened your mental equilibrium. Think about the relief of a calmer digestive system, fewer random aches and pains, and a general sense that you are more in control of your health destiny. These are the kinds of outcomes a vagus-focused approach can deliver. It's not a magic cure-all, but it *is* a way to unlock your body's innate capacity to heal and maintain balance – a capacity that often gets hampered by modern stress and lifestyle.

In closing, the vagus nerve is your body's secret to self-healing, and living a "vagus lifestyle" means embracing daily habits that keep this healing pathway switched on. The chapters to come will guide you through that process, step by step. By the end of this book, you will have built your own personalized routine of vagus-boosting practices. This routine will be your toolkit to sleep better, heal better, and in all likelihood, live longer and more vibrantly. You'll not only add years to your life, but add life to your years – enjoying a greater healthspan where you feel energetic, balanced, and truly alive.

Get ready to discover just how powerful these "small" daily actions can be. Armed with knowledge and inspired by real results, you are about to embark on a journey to tune your nervous system for optimal health. The vagus nerve may have been behind the scenes until now, but as you shine a light on it and start living the vagus lifestyle, you'll find that this humble nerve could indeed be the key to unlocking your healthiest, happiest self. Let's begin this transformation – one breath, one habit at a time – and watch your body's natural healing power flourish.

# Chapter 2

# From Fight-or-Flight to Rest-and-Digest – Taming Stress Through Your Vagus Nerve

## The Physiology of Calm

When life throws a curveball – a near car accident, an angry email, or any sudden scare – your body's "fight-or-flight" system kicks in. Heart pounding, muscles tensing, breath quickening: this is the sympathetic nervous system revving you up to face danger. It's like a gas pedal for survival, flooding your body with adrenaline and alertness. But just as crucial is the brake pedal: the parasympathetic nervous system, often called the "rest-and-digest" mode, which helps restore calm once the threat passes. At the center of this calming system is the vagus nerve – a long, wandering nerve that acts as an off-switch for stress. In a tug-of-war between stress and serenity, the vagus nerve tips the balance toward relaxation. Under stress, your sympathetic nerves fire up an alarm state; activating the vagus, however, counteracts that alarm, slowing the racing heart and easing tense muscles so you can return to baseline.

The vagus nerve is often referred to as the body's "chill out" command center – and for good reason. This nerve originates in the brainstem and wanders throughout the body, branching out to your heart, lungs, stomach, intestines, and more. Because it plugs into so many organs, it can send a wave of calm through multiple systems at once. Imagine your body as an orchestra of organs: during stress, the sympathetic system is like a frantic conductor speeding up the tempo. The vagus nerve steps in as the gentle maestro that slows the music back down. When the vagus is activated, it triggers the release of neurotransmitters that essentially tell your body "All is well." For example, the vagus nerve releases acetylcholine – a chemical messenger that signals your heart's pacemaker to slow down, dropping your heart rate and blood pressure. Your breathing naturally deepens and slows, digestion resumes, and blood flow returns to organs that were on pause during the alarm phase. In essence, turning on the vagus nerve creates a wave of calm that washes over you from head to toe.

This dynamic is part of our evolutionary design. The fight-or-flight response served our ancestors in life-or-death moments, but it's meant to be temporary – our bodies aren't built to stay in emergency mode forever. "States of threat are not sustainable long-term—we literally fall apart mentally and physically," one overview explains. Our built-in balancing mechanism is the vagus nerve: as soon as immediate danger passes, vagal signals kick in to shut off the stress response and bring the body back to a state of safety and recovery. In simple terms, the vagus nerve is the switch that flips the nervous system from high alert back to healing mode.

Physiologically, what does this calm state look like? Once the vagus engages, your racing heartbeat slows to a gentle rhythm, blood pressure lowers, and breathing becomes slow and even. Neurotransmitters and hormones associated with relaxation (like acetylcholine and serotonin) increase, while stress hormones like cortisol and adrenaline drop. You might even feel a sigh of relief or your stomach unclench – that's the parasympathetic influence easing both mind and body. This vagal activation isn't just about feeling relaxed in the moment; it has protective health benefits too. Research shows that a strong vagus response (sometimes called high vagal tone) is linked to a lower resting heart rate, healthy digestion, and even a more robust immune system. In contrast, when the vagus nerve's activity is low, people tend to be more prone to anxiety, have a harder time recovering from stress, and may experience issues like elevated blood pressure or inflammation. The key takeaway: your vagus nerve is the physiological command center of calm. By turning off the body's alarm and activating "rest-and-digest" functions, it restores equilibrium and helps you literally *relax from the inside out.*

In summary, the vagus nerve serves as a vital gearshift between stress and peace. It helps turn fight-or-flight into rest-and-digest by sending calming signals that override the stress response. Your pounding heart slows, tense muscles loosen, and a sense of safety returns as the vagus nerve does its job. Understanding this physiology of calm isn't just science trivia – it's empowering. It means that by learning to engage your vagus nerve, you hold a built-in switch to tame stress and coax your body back into balance whenever life pushes you into overdrive.

## Case Study – Overcoming Anxiety Naturally

Let's bring this science to life with a real-world example. Meet Maya, a 35-year-old project manager at a busy marketing firm. For years, Maya lived in a near-constant state of stress. Juggling client deadlines and long hours, she would wake up with her heart already racing. By the time she got to work, even minor problems – a tense meeting or a late email – sent her into full anxiety mode. Her chest tightened and pulse pounded in her ears, classic signs of her fight-or-flight response running rampant. In the evenings, Maya found it impossible to "turn off" and relax. She often lay in bed exhausted yet unable to sleep, her mind and body still stuck on high alert. Over time, this chronic stress started to take a toll. Maya's blood pressure crept upward and she experienced frequent tension headaches and digestive upset. She felt trapped in a cycle of anxiety that she couldn't control.

Everything began to change when Maya learned about engaging her vagus nerve. Initially, it was a recommendation from her doctor, who noticed her blood pressure was borderline high. Rather than immediately resort to medication, her doctor suggested she try some natural stress-reduction techniques – specifically, deep belly breathing exercises and mindfulness meditation – to activate her parasympathetic nervous system (with the vagus nerve as the key player). Skeptical but desperate for relief, Maya decided to give it a shot. She started simple: each morning before diving into work, she sat on her couch with one hand on her belly and practiced slow diaphragmatic breathing. Inhale for a count of 5… exhale for a count of 8… letting her belly rise and fall with each breath. The first few times, her mind raced and it felt almost too simple to be effective. But she noticed that during those minutes of focusing on breathing, her heart rate actually began to steady and a sense of quietude crept in.

Encouraged, Maya began using this belly breathing technique whenever she felt panic build – before a big meeting, sitting in her car after a stressful commute, even in the bathroom during a particularly overwhelming day. She also incorporated mini "vagus nerve breaks" into her routine. At lunch, she'd take a 5-minute walk around the block, breathing deeply and intentionally. In the evenings, she tried a guided mindfulness meditation to wind down, often involving a body scan and slow breathing to signal safety to her body. At first, the effects were subtle. She still had anxious moments, but she felt a little more *in control* – as if she had a hand on that internal dimmer switch, able to turn down the intensity of her body's stress alarm. The real payoff came after a few weeks of consistent practice. One afternoon, Maya was stuck in traffic when another driver cut her off, a situation that would previously have sent her into a furious stress response. This time, she noticed her hands unclenching more quickly. She automatically took a few slow, deep breaths (something that had become almost second nature), and to her surprise, her racing heart settled much faster than before. "It was like I flipped a calm switch inside," she later described to a friend.

Over the next couple of months, Maya's life transformed in concrete ways. Her coworkers remarked that she seemed "more relaxed" and handled last-minute crises at work with a new sense of composure. Instead of immediately panicking when a stressful event hit, she instinctively started engaging her vagus nerve – sometimes by taking a quiet moment to breathe deeply, other times by humming softly to herself between meetings (she'd learned that the vibrations of humming can stimulate vagal activity, and besides, it made her feel soothed). Maya's sleep improved as well. With a nightly breathing and meditation routine, she found it easier to drift off, and she slept more soundly. No longer jolting awake at 3 AM with her mind racing, she awoke more refreshed. Perhaps most impressively, at her next medical check-up, her doctor noted that Maya's blood pressure had dropped from the high end of normal to a much healthier range. Maya herself was astonished – she hadn't changed her diet or exercise drastically, but by managing her stress through vagus nerve activation, her body was literally responding with improved vital signs. (This isn't magic; in fact, studies have shown that practicing slow, deep breathing for just a few minutes a day can lower blood pressure by activating vagal relaxation reflexes.)

Maya's story demonstrates the real-world impact of vagus-centered stress management. She went from feeling like a helpless passenger on a wild rollercoaster of stress, to being an active driver who could apply the brakes. Instead of spiraling into panic during a tough day, she learned to recognize the early signs of her fight-or-flight kicking in – the quickened pulse, the anxious tightness in her chest – and then consciously engage her vagus nerve to counteract it. Deep belly breathing became her go-to tool to quell panic attacks before they took hold. By exhaling slowly and extending her out-breath, she was tapping into the vagal signals that tell the brain and heart to calm down. And it paid off: she felt *calmer*, gained confidence that she could handle stress, and even saw measurable health improvements like better sleep and steadier blood pressure.

This case might sound familiar to anyone who has dealt with chronic stress or anxiety. The techniques Maya used are simple – no special equipment, nothing costly – but their effects were profound because they target the body's natural calming pathway. Her journey underscores a hopeful message: even if you're someone who feels constantly anxious or "wired," you can learn to shift your body into a calmer state by engaging the vagus nerve. It takes practice and patience, as it did for Maya, but the results can be life-changing. For Maya, overcoming anxiety naturally wasn't about willpower or "just relaxing" – it was about working with her physiology. By regularly practicing vagus-activating habits, she essentially trained her nervous system to not overreact to everyday stressors. Her story shows what's possible for anyone looking to tame stress: with the vagus nerve as an ally, you can break out of fight-or-flight and find your way to steady ground again.

## Insights from Stress Experts

What do neuroscientists, psychologists, and health experts have to say about this vagus-stress connection? In a word: *plenty*. Modern research is confirming that many of the activities we associate with relaxation owe much of their power to the vagus nerve. In fact, experts often note that the reason practices like deep breathing, meditation, gentle yoga, or massage feel so calming is that they stimulate vagal activity, which in turn slows our physiology from anxious to tranquil. *"It turns out that many of the activities that we associate with calmness—things like deep breathing, meditation, massage and even the experience of awe—effect changes in the brain, in part, through increasing vagus nerve activity,"* explains Dr. Vernon Williams, a neurologist who studies mind-body health. In other words, your serene yoga class or your quiet time breathing isn't "just in your head" – it creates real, measurable shifts in your biology via the vagus nerve. When you take slow breaths or get a gentle massage, you are literally nudging your body's nerves toward a state of calm. The vagus nerve sends signals that counteract the stress response, and this has been observed in scientific studies. One Scientific American report put it succinctly: when stress signals get excessive, *"the brain sends messages down the vagus to activate the countervailing 'rest-and-digest' system,"* releasing acetylcholine in the heart to reduce heart rate and blood pressure and relax the body. The science backs up what we instinctively feel – those calming activities truly work on a physiological level.

Clinicians are leveraging these insights in practice, teaching patients how to harness the vagus nerve for better stress management. For example, Dr. Yufang Lin, an integrative medicine physician at the Cleveland Clinic, often coaches her patients in techniques like breathing exercises, meditation, and even biofeedback to strengthen their vagal response. She highlights that consistency is key. *"When you repeat these activities over time, you increase heart rate variability and strengthen your vagus nerve function,"* Dr. Lin says. *"Then, the next time your sympathetic nervous system responds to a trigger, you can recover faster.".* Heart Rate Variability (HRV) is a metric researchers use as a proxy for vagal tone – essentially, how flexibly your heart can toggle between stress and relaxation. Higher HRV means a more resilient, vagus-influenced heart, and Dr. Lin's point is that regularly engaging in calming practices boosts this resilience. Her experience echoes a growing consensus in the medical community: patients who cultivate strong vagal tone (through mind-body practices like slow breathing, mindfulness, or gentle exercise) often see reductions in anxiety and improvements in how they handle stress day-to-day. In therapy settings, psychologists might employ HRV biofeedback, where patients learn to control their breath and heart rhythms while watching feedback monitors. This technique essentially trains you to activate your vagus nerve on command. Studies show it can significantly reduce symptoms of anxiety by teaching the body to self-calm more efficiently. It's a high-tech validation of an age-old idea: by controlling our breath and engaging the parasympathetic system, we gain control over our stress.

Notably, many experts emphasize that simple habits can have profound effects. You don't necessarily need expensive devices or complex interventions to tap into vagal calming. Dr. Vernon Williams (mentioned above) and others point to everyday actions – breathing deeply, humming, meditating, gentle yoga – as vagus stimulators that they recommend widely. Tracye Freeman Valentine, a clinical therapist, adds that even vocal exercises can help: *"Deep and slow breathing activates the vagus nerve and leads to a reduction in anxiety and stress responses,"* she notes, and using techniques like extending the exhale or humming can further calm an agitated nervous system. In fact, humming or singing is often suggested by therapists because the vibrations in the throat directly engage branches of the vagus nerve, signaling the body to relax. You might have noticed you naturally hum to soothe yourself – now science explains why. Similarly, Dr. Stephen Porges, a neuroscientist famous for formulating the Polyvagal Theory, has illuminated how feeling safe (versus threatened) is largely mediated by vagal activity. According to Porges, when our vagus nerve is active, it promotes a physiological state of safety and social connection; when it's not, we're more prone to anxiety and defensive reactions. This theory has influenced trauma therapists to incorporate vagal activation (through breathing, grounding exercises, etc.) as a way to help patients regain a sense of safety after stress.

From a research standpoint, evidence for the vagus-stress link is robust and growing. A 2023 meta-analysis of clinical trials found that deliberate breathwork interventions were associated with significantly lower levels of stress and anxiety in participants compared to those who did nothing special. The findings suggest that learning to slow down your breathing and engage the parasympathetic system isn't just relaxing in the moment – it can tangibly improve mental health outcomes. Another line of research has examined practices like meditation and found they can increase vagal tone over time, which correlates with improved emotional regulation and even cognitive benefits. Neuroscientists using brain imaging have observed that when people practice mindfulness or slow breathing, there's increased activity in brain regions that regulate emotions and a corresponding increase in parasympathetic (vagal) signals to the heart. This blend of clinical wisdom and scientific data should be reassuring: the simple exercises that make you feel calm are backed by biology. When your psychologist or doctor advises deep breathing or meditation, it's not a vague platitude – it's a targeted technique to activate your vagus nerve, grounded in research.

Perhaps one of the most encouraging expert insights is how *empowering* this vagal connection can be. As Dr. Lin noted, strengthening your vagal response gives you a buffer against future stressors – a form of stress inoculation. If you regularly practice engaging your vagus nerve, it's like training a muscle; over time, your body learns to snap into calm more easily. This means that even if you can't change the stressful circumstances around you, you *can* change how your body reacts. That concept has gained mainstream attention, with major hospitals (Massachusetts General, Cedars-Sinai, etc.) educating patients on vagus nerve stimulation techniques as adjunct therapy for anxiety, PTSD, and inflammatory conditions. The consensus from experts is clear: nurturing your vagus nerve is a science-backed way to tame stress. By incorporating vagal-boosting habits into daily life, you're not just following a wellness trend – you're tuning your nervous system for better health and resilience. As research continues, we'll likely see even more innovative uses of vagus nerve stimulation in medicine. But you don't have to wait for the future – the knowledge is already here, and the practices are available to everyone right now.

## Daily Calm-Down Techniques

Armed with the understanding that activating your vagus nerve can bring you back to calm, the next step is knowing *how* to do it. Fortunately, you don't need any fancy equipment or intensive training to tap into your vagal "calm switch." In fact, some of the most effective techniques are downright simple and can be done anytime, anywhere. Below is a toolbox of daily calm-down techniques – practical exercises that stimulate your vagus nerve and help manage stress in the moment. Try incorporating these into your routine. With regular practice, they can become healthy habits that make engaging your body's relaxation response almost second nature.

- **Deep Diaphragmatic Breathing:** The fastest way to engage your vagus nerve is through your breath. Most of us tend to take shallow "chest breaths" when anxious, but here you will do the opposite: breathe deeply into your belly. *How to do it:* Sit or stand comfortably and place one hand on your abdomen. Inhale slowly through your nose for a count of about 6, feeling your belly expand, then exhale gently through your mouth for a count of about 8, fully emptying your lungs. (If the count of 6 and 8 feels too long, start with 4 and 6 seconds, then work up.) The key is to make your exhale longer than your inhale – that prolonged exhalation especially activates the vagus nerve and sends signals of calm to your heart and brain. As you breathe, try to focus only on the sensation of the air flowing and your hand rising and falling on your belly. Even a few minutes of deep belly breathing can keep your vagus nerve active, essentially telling your nervous system that it's okay to relax. Many people find that 5 minutes of diaphragmatic breathing in the morning sets a peaceful tone for the day, and doing it again during moments of tension (for example, before a presentation or after an argument) quickly helps steady the nerves. This technique is so effective that cardiologists note it can sometimes lower blood pressure as much as medication over time – truly a powerhouse habit for stress relief.

- **Mindfulness Meditation Breaks:** Carving out short meditation breaks can significantly dial down stress by heightening vagal activity. Meditation and mindfulness practices work by calming the mind and, in turn, calming the body – partly via the vagus nerve's influence. Even a brief 5–10 minute meditation can activate your parasympathetic nervous system. *How to do it:* Find a quiet spot (even your parked car or a bathroom stall can work in a pinch). Close your eyes and bring your attention to the present moment. You might focus on your breath (as in the exercise above) or do a quick body scan, observing sensations from head to toe. If your mind wanders – which it will – gently bring your focus back to your breathing or your body, without self-judgment. This simple practice lowers heart rate and blood pressure, indicating a shift toward relaxation. *"Meditation and mindfulness not only lower your heart rate, but they also reduce blood pressure levels,"* notes Dr. Mitzi Gonzales, a neuropsychologist, underscoring how these mental exercises translate into physical calm. To get the most benefit, integrate mini-meditation pauses into your day. For example, you might take 5 minutes at lunchtime to sit quietly and breathe, or do a short guided meditation using a smartphone app after work to transition into a relaxed evening. Over time, these meditation breaks strengthen your vagal tone – essentially exercising your "calm muscle" – and you may notice that stressors don't rattle you as much as they once did.

- **Humming, Singing, and Chanting:** It might sound surprising, but using your voice can be a direct route to stimulating the vagus nerve. The act of humming or softly singing causes vibrations in your throat that activate the vagal fibers running to your vocal cords and throat. This is why activities like chanting "Om" in yoga or singing in the shower can leave you feeling blissfully relaxed. *How to do it:* You can hum your favorite tune, chant a soothing syllable (like "om" or even a simple "mmm" sound), or sing along to music in a gentle tone. The key is the vibration and the elongated exhale that naturally occurs when you hum or sing a phrase. For instance, take a comfortable breath in, then hum as you exhale slowly; feel the buzz in your throat and chest. That vibration is tickling the vagus nerve. Therapists have noted that *"humming, singing, or even gargling can stimulate the vagus nerve, increasing heart rate variability and vagal tone,"* which are signs of a relaxed, resilient nervous system. Even just 30 seconds of humming a lullaby or chanting can induce a feeling of tranquility. Some people make a habit of humming whenever they feel stressed – say, during a tough commute or while doing chores – as a way to self-soothe. Don't worry if you're out of tune; this isn't about performance, but about physical effect. If you prefer, try gentle chanting: you might repeat a calming word or mantra in a low, drawn-out voice. The content of what you sing or say doesn't matter as much as the act of creating a resonant sound. Experiment to see what kind of sound makes you feel most calm. You may be pleasantly surprised at how quickly a bit of humming can melt away tension (it's one reason people instinctively hum or sing to themselves when nervous).

- **Self-Massage and Pressure Points:** Physical touch, especially around certain areas of the body, can prompt a vagus nerve response and help release stress. While a professional massage is wonderful, you can also reap benefits from simple self-massage techniques focused on the neck, shoulders, and feet – regions that have lots of nerve endings connected to the vagus pathways. *How to do it:* One easy exercise is a neck massage. Gently rub the sides of your neck (where your carotid arteries are) with slow, circular motions. You're near the vagus nerve's path there, and gentle pressure can stimulate it. Likewise, you can massage the back of your neck and shoulders, kneading out tension – this not only loosens tight muscles but also promotes a parasympathetic response. Another approach is foot reflexology. Using your thumbs, apply gentle pressure to the soles of your feet and massage in slow strokes. Amazingly, studies have shown that a foot massage can boost vagal activity and even *lower blood pressure* by nudging your body toward relaxation. Even if the science weren't there, most people agree that a foot rub or shoulder rub just makes them feel more at ease – now we know it's partly due to vagus nerve activation. You can also try a facial or scalp massage: lightly massaging your scalp, temples, or even doing a bit of ear massage (the outer ear has a branch of the vagus nerve) can be calming. Some individuals practice a technique of gently massaging the tragus (that small triangular part in front of your ear canal) which can stimulate the auricular branch of the vagus nerve – but only use light pressure and stop if you feel discomfort. The general rule with vagus-focused massage is to keep it gentle and pleasant. Unlike deep tissue massage that can sometimes be painful (and ironically trigger a stress response), *gentle touch* is best for activating the calming nerves. Try ending your day with a few minutes of self-massage on your neck or feet as part of a wind-down routine. It's a simple ritual that tells your body it's okay to relax now.

In addition to these techniques, there are other vagus-friendly habits you can weave into daily life. Mild exercise is one – activities like yoga, tai chi, or even a relaxed walk can increase vagal tone and reduce stress. Laughing with a friend, listening to soothing music, or practicing gratitude are also indirect ways to engage the parasympathetic system. Even cold water splashes on your face or ending a shower with a brief cool rinse can activate the "dive reflex," stimulating the vagus nerve and calming you down (think of how a splash of cool water can sometimes stop panic in its tracks). The toolbox is full of options, and you can choose what resonates most with you.

The most important part is to make these practices a habit. The vagus nerve responds to consistent nurturing. Consider starting your morning with 5 minutes of deep breathing or a short meditation to set a calm baseline. During the day, use quick vagus activators as needed – perhaps humming to yourself in the car, or doing a few neck stretches and self-massage breaks during work. In the evening, unwind with another breathing session or a warm tea while humming a little tune. These might seem like small actions, but their cumulative effect is powerful. Over time, you're effectively training your nervous system to know how to relax. It's like exercising a muscle: repetition builds strength. *"When you repeat these activities over time, you… strengthen your vagus nerve function,"* as Dr. Lin noted, which means the next time you encounter a stressful trigger, your body can recover its calm more quickly. By routinely activating this "calm switch," you'll likely find that you become more resilient – stress still happens, but it doesn't overwhelm you as easily. Instead, you'll have confidence that your body has a built-in way to regain equilibrium.

In embracing these daily vagus nerve habits, you're adopting what we might call the "Vagus Lifestyle." It's a lifestyle where managing stress becomes a proactive daily practice, not an afterthought. Little by little, breath by breath, hum by hum, you are teaching your body how to shift from fight-or-flight to rest-and-digest. The payoff is a life lived with a greater sense of ease, better sleep, a stronger immune system, and an empowered awareness that you hold the reins to your own stress responses. So take a deep breath – literally – and know that each time you do, you're tapping into your body's natural healing power to create calm from within. Your vagus nerve is waiting to be your ally in health, all it needs is a bit of daily attention. By integrating these simple practices, you're well on your way to living longer, sleeping better, and fortifying your body's innate resilience, one calming habit at a time.

# Chapter 3

## Rest and Restore – Harnessing the Vagus Nerve for Better Sleep

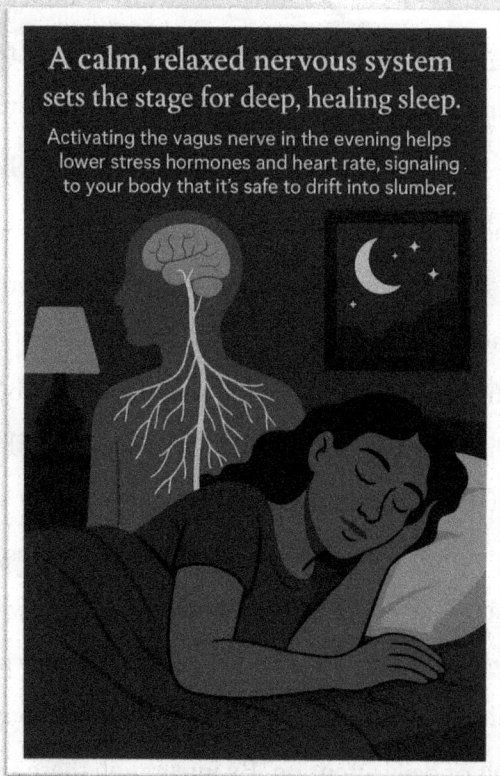

A calm, relaxed nervous system sets the stage for deep, healing sleep.

Activating the vagus nerve in the evening helps lower stress hormones and heart rate, signaling to your body that it's safe to drift into slumber.

## The Vagus–Sleep Connection

A good night's rest isn't just about having a comfy bed – it starts with a relaxed nervous system. The vagus nerve, known as the body's "rest and digest" highway, plays a critical role in shifting our physiology into sleep mode. In fact, the parasympathetic nervous system (largely driven by the vagus nerve) must be activated for us to achieve quality sleep. When evening comes and the vagus nerve is gently stimulated, it triggers a cascade of calming effects: heart rate slows, blood pressure eases down, and stress hormones like cortisol dip to low levels. This internal signal tells your body it's safe to wind down, creating the ideal conditions for falling asleep.

Scientific research backs up this vagus–sleep connection. Vagus nerve activation can reduce stress, lower cortisol levels, and improve heart rate variability (HRV) – all linked to deeper, more restorative sleep and healthy REM cycles. In other words, a higher "vagal tone" (a strong, responsive vagus nerve) helps you transition into the relaxed state needed for deep sleep. People with high vagal tone tend to have lower resting heart rates and a more balanced nervous system, which translates into smoother shifts from wakefulness into sleep. They often experience more refreshing sleep and even improvements in REM sleep quality. REM sleep – the dream-rich stage important for memory and mood – can be enhanced when the vagus nerve is functioning well, because the body isn't trapped in fight-or-flight mode.

Conversely, chronic stress or low vagal activity can wreak havoc on your sleep. If your vagus nerve isn't doing its job of calming you down, the sympathetic "fight or flight" system stays dominant, keeping your body on high alert at night. High stress means high cortisol and adrenaline at times when they should be lowest, and the result can be insomnia: racing thoughts, a pounding heart, and restless nights.

Research has shown that vagus nerve dysfunction or low vagal tone can disrupt normal sleep patterns, contributing to insomnia, fragmented sleep, and even conditions like sleep apnea. For example, obstructive sleep apnea – in which breathing repeatedly stops during sleep – has been linked in part to autonomic nervous system imbalances. Indeed, sleep specialists note that activating the calming vagus pathway is essential to counteract stress-related insomnia and some features of sleep apnea. It's a scientific reassurance that "toning" your vagus nerve isn't just wellness lingo: it can directly translate to falling asleep faster and sleeping more soundly.

Understanding this mind-body link gives us a powerful insight: by caring for and stimulating our vagus nerve (through simple daily habits), we are essentially telling our brain and body, "It's okay to let go." You are engaging your built-in "relaxation response", which renowned cardiologist Dr. Herbert Benson described as the opposite of the stress response. Tapping into that response via the vagus nerve at bedtime flips the switch from alertness to relaxation. Heart rate dips, breathing becomes slow and steady, and even your pupils constrict (letting in less light) as the vagus nerve engages the parasympathetic system to help you ease into sleep. This is why anything that relaxes your vagus nerve in the evening – whether it's deep breathing, a mindfulness practice, or gentle stretching – can pay huge dividends when your head hits the pillow.

In short, the vagus–sleep connection is the science of safety and restoration. When your brain perceives safety, it allows sleep; when your vagus nerve signals "all clear," your body enters a pre-sleep calm. By contrast, if your inner alarm systems are ringing (due to stress, anxiety, or low vagal tone), sleep can be elusive. The encouraging news is that you can strengthen this connection. Building vagal tone through daily habits effectively gives you a "sleep switch" to flip at night – sending you into deep rest mode more readily. Throughout the rest of this chapter, we'll explore exactly how to do that, from inspiring real-life examples to expert-backed tips and step-by-step bedtime rituals.

## Case Study – Beating Insomnia Naturally

Let's meet Mark, a 46-year-old accountant and father of two, who for years felt trapped in a cycle of insomnia. Mark would collapse into bed exhausted each night, only to find his mind racing and his body unable to relax. He often resorted to prescription sleeping pills, which left him groggy, or a couple of glasses of wine, which only fractured his sleep further. Over time, chronic lack of sleep made his days feel like wading through mud – he was irritable, unfocused at work, and dependent on caffeine to get by. Yet, like so many, Mark was hesitant about long-term pill use and yearned for a natural solution to his sleeplessness.

Everything changed when Mark learned about the vagus nerve and its role in relaxation. Skeptical but hopeful, he decided to try a new bedtime routine that focused on vagus-friendly habits instead of pills. First, he made a rule to turn off all screens at least an hour before bed. This meant shutting down his laptop, silencing work emails, and trading the glare of the TV for the soft glow of a book. This wasn't easy at first – Netflix had been his go-to wind-down. But Mark soon found that avoiding screens helped quiet his mind. Without the flood of blue light and information, his brain started producing melatonin on cue and his nervous system began to slow down in the evenings. He would dim the lights in the house and even started listening to quiet, soothing music as he put the kids to bed – a signal to his body that nighttime was for unwinding.

Next, Mark introduced a breathing exercise into his nightly regimen. He had read about the famous 4-7-8 deep breathing method – inhaling for 4 seconds, holding for 7, and exhaling for 8 – which is known to activate the vagus nerve and trigger a relaxation response. It felt a bit odd at first, counting out seconds in the dark, but he stuck with it. Every night, after getting into his pajamas, Mark would sit up in bed and do 10 minutes of 4-7-8 breathing. As he inhaled deeply into his belly and then released a long, slow exhale, he could actually feel a wave of calm wash over him. His heart rate slowed and the tension in his shoulders melted away. This breathing technique works by *lengthening the exhale*, which specifically stimulates the vagus nerve and tells the brain to switch into "rest" mode. In Mark's case, after a week of consistent practice, he noticed that as soon as he started his breathing ritual, his body seemed to know *"ah, it's time to sleep."* He described it as a natural sedative, without any medication – just breath. (Notably, scientific studies have shown that slow, diaphragmatic breathing can indeed calm the nervous system: it lowers blood pressure and signals the vagus nerve to induce relaxation.)

Perhaps the most surprising trick in Mark's new arsenal was an odd but effective cold therapy hack. One of his friends had sent him an article about using an ice pack on the chest or neck to help with insomnia. The idea sounded like Internet lore, but it actually has some scientific basis: exposing the body to cold can activate the vagus nerve via the "diving reflex," rapidly slowing the heart rate and promoting calm. Determined to sleep better, Mark gave it a try. After his breathing exercise, he would place a small ice pack over the center of his chest (wrapped in a thin cloth) for a minute or two as he lay in bed. The cold sensation was bracing, but he noticed an interesting effect – it was as if a "switch" flipped in his body, triggering a heavy relaxation. In fact, experts say that stimulating the vagus nerve with a cold pack at bedtime can indeed spur the parasympathetic system into action, making you feel more relaxed. One small study found that applying cold to the neck area slowed down people's heart rates and increased vagal activity (a marker of relaxation). True to this, Mark found that after a brief chilly press on his chest, his previously racing heartbeat would steady into a calm rhythm. His body got the message: it's time to rest.

Mark also incorporated a few other quirky but effective habits. He started doing a simple yoga pose, "legs up the wall," each night for a couple of minutes – lying on his back with legs vertically resting on the wall. This gentle inversion is known to stimulate the vagus nerve and drain tension. Sometimes he would also do Child's Pose, kneeling and curling forward with arms extended, which always released low back stress. These stretches further nudged his body toward relaxation, and Mark found the slow breathing and gentle pressure in these poses deeply soothing.

The transformation didn't happen overnight, but over several weeks, Mark's sleepless nights turned into sound slumbers. By sticking to his vagus-focused routine – no screens, deep breathing, a bit of cold therapy, and stretches – he retrained his nervous system. The results were remarkable: he fell asleep faster, without the hour of tossing and turning that used to plague him, and he stayed asleep longer. If he did wake briefly, he was able to do a few 4-7-8 breaths and drift back to sleep, rather than spiraling into panic about being awake. His wife remarked that he even *looked* calmer in the evenings, no longer pacing around in a wired state. And each morning, Mark woke up clear-headed and refreshed instead of groggy. The newfound energy in his days felt like a superpower. He could concentrate at work again and had patience to play with his kids after work, all thanks to finally sleeping well.

Mark's journey from frazzled insomniac to well-rested and pill-free is a powerful example of how leveraging vagus nerve habits can break the vicious cycle of insomnia. He proved that even long-time poor sleepers can reclaim peaceful nights by using the body's own calming mechanisms. No longer dependent on pills or alcohol, Mark's story shows that beating insomnia naturally is possible – and often, it's about consistency with a few simple practices. His routine might sound unique, but it's rooted in solid principles of sleep science and nervous system regulation. If you identified with Mark's "racing mind at 2 A.M." struggles, take heart: your vagus nerve could be the secret key to calming your mind and finally getting the restorative sleep you crave.

## Expert Sleep Tips

What do sleep medicine specialists and neurologists say about harnessing the vagus nerve for better sleep? In a nutshell, they agree: activating the body's relaxation response at night is one of the best things you can do for your sleep quality. Dr. Stefanie N. Howell, a neurologist who has researched sleep-wake disorders, explains that engaging the vagus nerve is so effective because it directly taps into the relaxation pathways in our brain and body. *"The relaxation effect is a major factor in why stimulating the vagus nerve can help with sleep,"* Dr. Howell notes, adding that there's evidence the vagus nerve is directly involved in regulating the brain's sleep-wake circuitry. In other words, techniques that calm your vagus nerve don't just make you *feel* relaxed – they may actually help synchronize the very networks in the brain that control when you sleep and wake. This expert insight gives a stamp of authority to our approach: the practices that make you say "ahh" in the evening (like deep breathing or meditation) are truly setting the neurological stage for quality sleep.

So, what specific tips do experts recommend to activate your parasympathetic (vagal) system at night? First on the list is maintaining a regular sleep schedule. Consistency – going to bed and waking up at the same time every day – helps the body's internal clock know when to naturally engage the vagus nerve and begin the nightly wind-down. Our bodies thrive on routine; a stable schedule trains your nervous system to predict when it's time to shift into rest mode. Many sleep doctors emphasize that irregular bedtimes can keep your system off-balance, whereas a regular routine is like a gentle coach for your vagal tone, nudging it to kick in each evening.

Another top tip is creating a wind-down ritual in the hour before sleep – a predictable sequence that tells your body "the day is done, it's time to relax." According to Dr. Howell and others, this ritual can include activities known to increase vagal activity and decrease fight-or-flight arousal. For example, doing a brief mindfulness meditation or gentle yoga session in the evening can send your vagus nerve a clear message to relax. Even just 5–10 minutes of quiet meditation (focusing on your breath or a calming image) is shown to increase vagal tone; over time, regular meditation literally trains your parasympathetic system to activate more readily. Some sleep experts advise their patients to pair this with soothing music – a strategy supported by research. In fact, a systematic review confirmed that listening to calming music positively influences the autonomic nervous system, increasing parasympathetic activity and heart rate variability (HRV) (a good thing for relaxation). This means putting on some soft classical or ambient music before bed isn't just mood-setting; it can physically shift your body into a more vagus-friendly state. Low, slow rhythms (around 60 beats per minute, like a resting heartbeat) tend to be most effective at encouraging your heart and breathing to slow down in tandem.

Experts also highlight the importance of reducing stimulation at night – which aligns with Mark's approach of cutting out screens. Bright lights, late-night work emails, or intense TV shows can keep your sympathetic nervous system (the alert, fight-or-flight side) in high gear, directly counteracting vagus nerve efforts. Dr. Adrian Pristas, a sleep medicine specialist, puts it bluntly: it's unrealistic to expect perfect sleep if you're "pressing on the gas and the brake at the same time." A calming pre-sleep environment is crucial. Dimming the lights, keeping the bedroom cool, and doing something relaxing (like light reading or taking a warm bath) all help coax your vagus nerve into dominance by bedtime. Some clinicians even suggest a digital curfew, such as "no electronics after 9 PM," to minimize mental stimulation and blue light exposure that can suppress your body's natural melatonin. By limiting these external stressors, you allow the vagus nerve's calming influence to shine through unopposed.

On a more high-tech front, there is intriguing clinical research on direct vagus nerve stimulation as a therapy for insomnia. Medical experts have been studying whether gentle electrical stimulation of the vagus nerve (through a device on the ear or implanted in the chest) can improve sleep in people with serious insomnia. The results so far are promising. A 2024 randomized clinical trial found that daily transcutaneous auricular vagus nerve stimulation (taVNS) significantly reduced insomnia severity, with participants sleeping better and scoring higher on sleep quality indices compared to a sham (placebo) treatment. These improvements were not fleeting – they were sustained even months after the 8-week stimulation protocol. Similarly, a narrative review in 2025 noted that although more research is needed, existing studies show taVNS can improve sleep quality and ease accompanying anxiety in insomnia patients. Sleep physicians point out that while we're not yet at the point of prescribing vagus nerve stimulators for every insomniac, these findings reinforce how pivotal the vagus nerve is in sleep regulation. They also underline a practical point: anything you do to manually stimulate your vagus nerve (even non-electrically, via breathing or cold or meditation) is tapping into the same system these therapies target. It's both empowering and exciting to realize that cutting-edge sleep medicine is, in a way, validating the age-old relaxation practices we can do on our own.

In summary, the expert advice boils down to a simple but profound idea: engage your body's natural relaxation response every night. Maintain consistency, have a wind-down routine, incorporate mind-body techniques like deep breathing, meditation or relaxing music – all these help activate your vagus nerve and quiet the stress responses that hinder sleep. By following these recommendations, you're essentially acting as your own sleep coach, compassionately guiding your physiology from a busy day into a peaceful night.

## Bedtime Rituals for Vagal Tone

Now it's time to put knowledge into practice. Here is a step-by-step guide to nightly habits that can immediately help you harness the power of the vagus nerve for better sleep. Think of this as your personalized "Rest and Restore" ritual – the last hour of your day will become a pro-vagus, pro-sleep routine. Each step is simple and backed by the principles we've discussed. You can mix and match what works for you, but doing several in combination will supercharge your vagal tone before bed. Let's dive in:

1. **Unplug and Set the Mood**: Power down your screens and dim the lights at least 30–60 minutes before bedtime. By turning off

the TV, computer, and smartphone, you're removing sources of mental stimulation and blue light that can keep your brain wired. This gives your vagus nerve a chance to assert the calm of the parasympathetic system without competition. Use this time to engage in quiet, relaxing activities instead – perhaps read a light book, write in a journal, or listen to soft music. Dimming lights (or using warm, low-level lamps) signals your brain that night is here, encouraging melatonin release and a natural relaxation response. Think of this step as creating a nest of safety: a cocoon of calm where your body and mind feel secure enough to let go. The vagus nerve loves a tranquil environment. By intentionally avoiding stressful content or work-related thoughts late at night, you prevent triggering the "fight or flight" reflex. In this peaceful atmosphere, your heart rate can start to slow and cortisol can fall, setting the stage for quality sleep.

2.  **Gentle Yoga or Stretching:** Engage in 10 minutes of gentle movement or yoga poses that promote relaxation. This is a physical way to signal to your body that wakeful activity is ending. Certain poses are especially effective at stimulating vagal tone. For example, Child's Pose – kneeling and bowing forward with arms extended – is a restorative pose that helps release tension in the back and neck and can activate the vagus nerve through slow, deep breathing in the folded position. Cat-Cow stretch (arching and rounding the back on hands and knees) is another beginner-friendly move that massages the spine and encourages diaphragmatic breathing. In fact, yoga poses that focus on

relaxation, such as Child's Pose or Cat-Cow, have been noted to activate the vagus nerve and ramp up the parasympathetic response. As you stretch or hold these poses, breathe slowly and mindfully. Incorporating mindfulness – for instance, focusing on the sensation of the stretch and the sound of your breath – enhances the calming effect. This little yoga session should feel pleasant and unhurried, not a workout. The goal is to loosen any physical tightness from your day (stress often lodges in our muscles) and to directly engage body-based calming signals. Even if you're not a "yoga person," simple stretches like rolling your shoulders, gently twisting your torso, or lying on your back and hugging your knees to your chest can stimulate vagus-rich areas and tell your nervous system it's time to unwind.

3. **Practice Deep Breathing (4-7-8 Method):** After stretching, transition into deep breathing exercises for another 5–10 minutes. Controlled breathing is one of the fastest ways to activate the vagus nerve and shift into a relaxed state. A highly recommended technique is the 4-7-8 breathing method, which Mark used in our case study. To do this, inhale through your nose for a count of 4, hold the breath for a count of 7, then exhale slowly through your mouth for a count of 8. This pattern forces you to prolong your exhale, and those long exhalations are key to stimulating vagal activity. As you exhale, imagine stress leaving your body with your breath. Deep breathing like this slows your heart rate and lowers blood pressure, telling every cell in your body that you are safe and can power down for the night. If 4-7-

8 is too advanced at first, you can try simpler belly breathing: inhale for 3 seconds, exhale for 6 seconds, then gradually lengthen it. The exact counts aren't magic – it's the principle of deep, slow, rhythmic breathing that matters. As you practice, you may notice a gentle tingling or wave of relaxation, which is a sign of the vagus nerve doing its job. Consistent nightly breathwork not only helps you feel calm in the moment, but over time it can increase your vagal tone overall, meaning your body becomes quicker to relax and recover from stress at all times. This is a habit that pays dividends in both nighttime sleep and daytime serenity.

4. **Humming, Chanting, or Praying:** This step might surprise you, but using your voice as a tool for relaxation can be incredibly effective. Humming, singing softly, or chanting "Om" out loud for a few minutes stimulates the vagus nerve through vibrations in your throat and vocal cords. You could put on a calming song and hum along, say a few prayers or affirmations in a low voice, or literally chant a long "Ommm" as done in meditation practices. It's not about musical talent at all – it's about the soothing vibration that resonates through your chest and throat, right where branches of the vagus nerve pass. Research shows that these kinds of vocal toning exercises increase heart rate variability and vagal tone, which are indicators of relaxation. In practical terms, humming or chanting creates a soothing effect that prepares your body for sleep. Many people find that after humming a lullaby or an "Om" for a minute or two, their mind feels quieter. You can combine this with step 3: for example, hum

on each extended exhale of your 4-7-8 breathing. Don't worry about how you sound – this is for your nervous system, not an audience. If you prefer not to make noise, even gently gargling water for 30 seconds can stimulate the vagus nerve similarly (an odd but therapist-approved trick!). The takeaway is to not overlook your voice as a built-in relaxation instrument. It's a fun, oddly satisfying addition to a bedtime routine that literally "vibrates" you into calm.

5. **Avoid Late Stimulants and Heavy Activity:** To support your vagus-focused rituals, it's important to minimize anything that would jolt your nervous system in the late evening. This means being mindful of caffeine, food, and exercise timing. Cut off caffeine at least 6–8 hours before bed (that 4 PM latte could still be in your system at midnight, keeping your heart rate up when you want it down). Similarly, avoid large meals or spicy food too close to bedtime – digestion uses the autonomic nervous system and a very full stomach might be counterproductive when you're trying to relax. If you're hungry, opt for a light snack (and perhaps something like chamomile tea which can encourage relaxation). Also consider the timing of strenuous exercise: a hard workout right before bed might leave you too pumped up, as adrenaline and sympathetic activity remain high for a while. Schedule vigorous exercise for earlier in the day if possible, and let the last hour be for gentler activities (like the yoga and breathing above). By avoiding stimulants – chemical or situational – you're removing obstacles that could overpower your vagus nerve's

calming efforts. Think of it this way: you wouldn't hit the accelerator when you intend to brake. Likewise, don't flood your body with stress signals when you intend to chill. In the last waking hour, aim to eliminate triggers of stress (intense debates, horror movies, work emails) and surround yourself with things that cue tranquility (a warm bath, lavender scent, quietude). This supportive environment allows your vagus nerve to do its job unhindered, guiding you into a restful night.

By implementing these rituals, you effectively make the last part of your day a vagus nerve tune-up. You're teaching your body a new pattern: evenings are for slowing down and activating healing mode. These habits may feel simple, but their impact is powerful because they align with our biology's natural design. Over time, as you practice unplugging, stretching, breathing, humming, and avoiding stimulants, you'll likely notice you fall asleep faster and sleep more soundly. Even more, you might find an overall improvement in your stress levels and mood, thanks to the cumulative boost in vagal tone. Remember, consistency is key – the vagus nerve strengthens like a muscle with regular use. Make your "Rest and Restore" ritual a non-negotiable part of your daily schedule, and soon it will become second nature.

In wrapping up this chapter, the message is an empowering one: your body possesses a natural healing power through the vagus nerve, and you can tap into it every single night. By consciously cultivating a vagus-friendly lifestyle – especially in how you approach sleep – you are not only going to bed, you are activating your body's built-in mechanisms for recovery and rejuvenation. Better sleep is just one reward. A stronger vagus response can also mean better digestion, a calmer mind, and even a more resilient immune system. It all interconnects. So as you turn off the lights and do your 4-7-8 breathing tonight, know that these small choices are cumulatively transforming your health. The vagus lifestyle is truly about gentle, daily practices that yield profound long-term benefits. With the simple rituals from this chapter, you're well on your way to living longer, sleeping better, and unleashing your body's natural healing power – all while enjoying the serenity of a good night's rest. Sweet dreams!

# Chapter 4

# The Anti-Inflammatory Reflex – Strengthening Immunity and Healing

Imagine your body has a hidden reflex, a built-in switch that tamps down inflammation whenever it flares up. This isn't science fiction – it's the power of the vagus nerve at work. In this chapter, we explore how the vagus nerve acts as an immune system ally, calming excessive inflammation through what scientists call the "cholinergic anti-inflammatory pathway." We'll see how this *internal anti-inflammatory reflex* helps prevent disease and aging by keeping our immune responses in balance. We'll also look at a real-world healing story, hear from experts on stress and immunity, and learn practical daily habits to engage your vagus nerve for better health. By the end, you'll understand why strengthening your vagus response can help you live longer, heal better, and feel more resilient every day.

## How the Vagus Fights Inflammation

Your vagus nerve isn't just for relaxation – it's also a frontline warrior against inflammation. Scientists have discovered a neural pathway in which signals traveling along the vagus nerve can dial down the release of inflammatory molecules (cytokines) in the body. This mechanism is often referred to as the "inflammatory reflex," and it works like an internal anti-inflammatory switch. When your body faces injury or infection, immune cells start pumping out cytokines (such as tumor necrosis factor, IL-1, IL-6) to fight off invaders. The vagus nerve monitors this activity and, if the inflammatory response starts raging out of control, it sends a calming signal – via the neurotransmitter acetylcholine – that tells immune cells (especially in organs like the spleen) to slow down the cytokine release. In essence, your brain, through the vagus nerve, can signal the immune system to "cool it," preventing an overreaction. This cholinergic pathway is a fascinating mind-body link: a nerve controlling the chemistry of your immune response in real time.

Why does this matter so much? Because chronic inflammation is a common thread in many serious diseases – from rheumatoid arthritis and inflammatory bowel disease to heart disease, diabetes, and even Alzheimer's. In fact, persistent low-grade inflammation is thought to accelerate aging itself (sometimes called "inflammaging") by causing constant wear-and-tear on organs and tissues. Excess inflammation doesn't just make you feel achy or tired; it actively damages cells and shortens lifespan if left unchecked. That's where a strong vagus nerve response becomes crucial. By keeping inflammatory cytokines in balance, a healthy vagal "anti-inflammatory reflex" allows your body to heal wounds and fight infections without collateral damage. It's the difference between a targeted immune strike and a scorched-earth approach. For example, if you cut your finger or catch the flu, you want your immune system to react *just enough* to heal, but not so much that it harms healthy tissue. The vagus nerve helps achieve that balance by preventing excessive inflammation that can cause pain, swelling, and tissue damage. This means less chance of acute injuries turning into chronic problems, and potentially even a slower aging process since your organs aren't constantly inflamed.

Think of the vagus nerve as an inflammation thermostat. When inflammation starts rising, the vagus nerve reflex kicks in to cool things down. This internal braking system was dramatically demonstrated in groundbreaking research by neurosurgeon Dr. Kevin Tracey. In his lab's experiments, stimulating the vagus nerve caused a notable drop in inflammatory cytokines like TNF-alpha, both in animals and humans. Tracey and colleagues showed that the brain-to-spleen vagus pathway can turn off inflammation at its source, preventing immune cells from overshooting the mark. This discovery of neural control over immunity revolutionized how scientists view the nervous system – it's not just a communication highway, but also a regulation system for the immune response. In short, the vagus nerve fights inflammation by acting as a built-in anti-inflammatory reflex. And keeping this reflex strong (through high "vagal tone") could be one of your best defenses against the chronic inflammation that underlies so many diseases.

## Case Study – Healing from Within

To see the vagus nerve's healing power in action, let's look at a real-world example. *Meet Sarah*, a 45-year-old woman living with rheumatoid arthritis, an autoimmune disease that causes painful joint inflammation. For years, Sarah managed her condition with medication, but she still experienced frequent flare-ups that left her joints swollen and stiff. Desperate for relief, she decided to try a different angle in addition to her doctor's treatments – she began daily vagus-oriented practices. Every morning, Sarah spent 15 minutes on deep breathing meditation and gentle yoga stretches. Every evening, she practiced relaxation techniques to wind down, sometimes including a short session of mindfulness or even humming to stimulate her vagus nerve. At first, she was skeptical that such simple habits could affect her immune system. But over the next few months, she noticed something remarkable: her flare-ups became less frequent and less severe. On many days, she woke up with little to no morning stiffness. Her pain levels dropped, and she found she needed anti-inflammatory medications less often. By integrating mind-body practices that toned her vagus nerve, Sarah essentially turned up her body's internal healing reflex. The result was *noticeable* – her immune system seemed less hyper-reactive, and she felt more in control of her disease.

Sarah's story mirrors what scientific studies are finding. In one clinical trial, patients with rheumatoid arthritis who completed an 8-week Mindfulness-Based Stress Reduction (MBSR) program (which combines meditation and gentle yoga) saw significant improvements in their symptoms. They reported less joint tenderness, pain, and morning stiffness compared to a control group. This improvement occurred even though objective lab markers (like C-reactive protein) didn't change much – suggesting that vagus-boosting activities were helping patients *experience* their condition differently, with lower perceived pain and inflammation. In other words, mind-body practices that activate the vagus nerve (such as meditation, slow breathing, and yoga) can translate into *measurable relief* for people with chronic inflammatory conditions. Patients often feel empowered by these techniques; instead of being at the mercy of their illness, they discover they can tap into the body's self-healing abilities.

Beyond lifestyle practices, doctors have even started using vagus nerve stimulation (VNS) therapy to fight inflammation in stubborn cases of disease. Imagine a tiny device, like a pacemaker, implanted under the skin that sends mild electrical pulses to your vagus nerve – essentially "dialing up" your anti-inflammatory reflex. In the case of rheumatoid arthritis, this once-futuristic idea is now a reality. A groundbreaking trial led by researchers at SetPoint Medical and other institutions tested an implanted vagus nerve stimulator in patients with severe, drug-resistant rheumatoid arthritis. The results were astonishing: vagus nerve stimulation drove down key inflammatory molecules by over 30%, including TNF-alpha, IL-1β, and IL-6, which are major drivers of arthritis flare-ups. Many patients experienced significant symptom relief and improved joint function as a result. One participant, who had endured years of pain and failed numerous medications, reported that after a few weeks of vagus stimulation, her rheumatoid arthritis symptoms had drastically diminished – she could open jars, walk longer distances, and resume activities she'd given up. This is a powerful illustration of "healing from within." By activating the vagus nerve's inflammatory reflex, the body can be prompted to heal itself in ways traditional drugs sometimes can't. While VNS therapy is still being refined and tested (in trials for arthritis, inflammatory bowel disease, and more), its success in cases like this shows just how much potential lies in enhancing our vagal tone. Whether through high-tech implants or simple daily habits, stimulating the vagus nerve can help tame chronic inflammation, allowing people like Sarah to reclaim their health and vitality.

## Expert Perspective on Immunity

The idea that a nerve can control inflammation might sound incredible, so let's hear from the experts who study this mind-body connection. Neuroimmunologists – scientists who research how the nervous and immune systems interact – have been at the forefront of this discovery. Dr. Kevin Tracey, a pioneer in this field, famously demonstrated that stress and inflammation are two sides of the same coin: stress hormones can send our immune system into overdrive or make it misfire, while vagus nerve signals can do the opposite, restoring balance. Chronic stress, for instance, floods the body with cortisol and adrenaline, which over time weakens immune defenses and promotes inflammation. Research shows that elevated stress hormones suppress key immune cells and skew cytokine levels, resulting in a *weaker immune response*. This is one reason people under long-term stress get sick more often – their immune "armor" is compromised. As Dr. Tracey and others explain, when you're stuck in fight-or-flight mode, your body thinks immediate survival is priority and downregulates longer-term healing and defense mechanisms.

Activating the vagus nerve flips that script. When you engage the vagal "brake," your body exits fight-or-flight and enters "rest-and-repair" mode, also known as the parasympathetic state. Stress hormones drop, heart rate slows, and blood pressure decreases. Internally, the vagus nerve is telling your spleen and other immune organs to calm down the cytokine storm. Dr. Luis Ulloa, a neuroimmunology researcher at Duke University, put it succinctly: *"Stimulating the vagus nerve neutralized the effects of stress and restored a balanced and healthy physiological state."* In other words, vagus activation is like an antidote to the immune-suppressing effects of stress. It not only relaxes your mind and body, but also lowers the inflammatory load by curbing excessive immune activity. This has huge implications for health. As one expert explained, many relaxation techniques (deep breathing, meditation, etc.) are essentially exercises in activating the vagus nerve, which in turn lowers stress-induced inflammation. By deliberately engaging this nerve through mindfulness or breathing, we can boost our resilience against infections and even improve how well vaccines work, according to emerging research.

Medical leaders are taking the vagus nerve *very* seriously. Dr. Tracey often talks about the "inflammatory reflex" as a natural target for therapy – a way to treat diseases by modulating nerves instead of just drugs. This concept has given birth to a new field called bioelectronic medicine, where devices are used to stimulate nerves (like the vagus) to treat disease. And it's not a far-off dream: vagus nerve stimulation is already an established therapy. In fact, since the 1990s, *over 100,000 people with epilepsy* have received implanted vagus stimulators to control seizures, and it's approved for treating depression as well. These patients walk around with an always-on vagus stimulator and generally tolerate it very well – a testament to how safe and integral this nerve is (common side effects are minor, like a slight hoarseness during stimulation). Now, researchers are piggybacking on that success to explore vagus stimulation for inflammatory and autoimmune conditions. Clinical trials are underway or in planning for diseases like Crohn's disease (a type of inflammatory bowel disease), lupus, arthritis, and even conditions like long COVID, where chronic inflammation and nervous system dysfunction are thought to play a role. Early results are promising. In small studies, vagus nerve stimulation has shown it can reduce inflammatory markers and symptoms in Crohn's patients and improve outcomes in difficult rheumatoid arthritis cases. A pilot study at Mount Sinai Hospital even found that daily non-invasive vagus stimulation (using ear clips) improved the health and energy levels of some long COVID patients who suffered from fatigue and inflammation.

What does this mean for you as a reader? It should be reassuring to know that the vagus-immunity connection isn't New Age woo-woo; it's grounded in serious science and medicine. When top neuroscientists and immunologists are publishing studies in journals like *Nature* and running clinical trials on vagus nerve stimulation, you can trust that this nerve is a key player in health. Experts emphasize that while we await more large-scale trials, there's enough evidence now to say chronic stress management and vagus activation are crucial for a strong immune system. As Dr. Tracey's work showed, the brain and immune system are in constant two-way communication. *Your thoughts and emotions can influence your immune cells via nerves.* That means techniques to reduce stress or directly stimulate the vagus (even simple deep breathing) truly can strengthen your immunity. Knowing this, doctors are increasingly advising patients to incorporate mind-body practices as part of comprehensive care. As one expert put it: *There's so much people can do on their own to support healing – when you activate your vagus nerve, you're basically tapping into your body's natural pharmacy of anti-inflammatories.* The medical community is excited about harnessing this, because it opens a new dimension of treatment: helping patients heal by modulating nerves and lifestyle, not just medications.

## Healing Habits for Your Vagus

By now it's clear that a toned vagus nerve can be a powerful healing force against inflammation and stress. The great news is that you don't need a surgical implant or a prescription to start engaging your vagus nerve. Here are some practical, everyday habits you can adopt to support your vagus nerve and immunity:

- **Move Your Body (Regular Moderate Exercise):** Physical activity is one of the simplest ways to boost vagal tone. When you exercise at a moderate intensity – like brisk walking, cycling, swimming, or dancing – you not only strengthen your heart and muscles, you also stimulate your parasympathetic nervous system. Regular exercise is linked with higher vagus activity and lower inflammation levels. In fact, people who stay active tend to have greater heart rate variability (a sign of strong vagal tone) and lower C-reactive protein (a blood marker of chronic inflammation). Think of exercise as training your "rest-and-digest" system to be more responsive. You don't have to run marathons; even 20-30 minutes of moderate activity a day is enough to send anti-inflammatory signals throughout your body. Over time, this habit can lower your baseline stress hormone levels and help your immune system remain balanced. Next time you break a sweat, remember: you're not just building muscle or burning calories, you're literally strengthening your body's anti-inflammatory reflex.

■ **Breathe and Relax (Mindful Breathing & Meditation):** Your breath is a direct dial to your vagus nerve. Slow, deep, diaphragmatic breathing – the kind where your belly expands on each inhale – activates vagal fibers in your diaphragm and lungs, which tells your brain to relax and triggers the parasympathetic response. Even a few minutes of such breathing can markedly increase vagal tone (often reflected by a calmer heart rate). Try techniques like 4-7-8 breathing (inhale for 4 counts, hold for 7, exhale for 8) or simply take long, slow breaths while focusing on the sensation of air in and out. You'll likely notice a sense of calm washing over you. That's your vagus nerve at work, reducing stress signals and inflammation. Beyond breathing, practices like meditation, mindfulness, and gentle yoga further engage the vagus nerve. These activities encourage the "relaxation response," lowering cortisol and adrenaline levels. Consistent meditation has been shown to improve heart rate variability and reduce inflammatory markers in some studies. Essentially, when you quiet your mind and body, you give your vagus nerve room to step on the brakes of your immune system – preventing unnecessary inflammatory spurts. Make it a habit to do at least one relaxing mind-body activity daily, whether it's breathing exercises in the morning, a short meditation break, or a calming yoga session at night. Over time, you'll build a more resilient vagal tone, meaning you react to daily stresses with less inflammation and tension.

- **Cool Off with Cold Exposure:** A bracing shot of cold can actually be good for your vagus nerve. Practices like ending your shower with a 30-second cold rinse, taking a quick cold plunge, or even splashing cold water on your face activate what's known as the "diving reflex." The sudden cold triggers vagus nerve pathways that slow your heart rate and ramp up parasympathetic activity (it's an ancient reflex to conserve energy in cold water). Many people find that regular brief cold exposure leaves them feeling invigorated yet calm – this is the vagus nerve response. What's more, emerging research suggests that cold stimulation can reduce inflammation by engaging vagal mechanisms. In studies, cooling the neck region (where the vagus nerve runs) led to increased heart rate variability and a drop in heart rate, indicating vagus activation. Some animal research even found that cold therapy tempered inflammatory responses via vagus pathways. You don't need an ice bath to get benefits; simply finishing your shower with cold water or dunking your face in cool water for 15 seconds can do the trick. It might be a bit uncomfortable at first, but that deep breath you instinctively take when the cold hits is activating your vagus nerve. Over time, you may notice improvements in your stress resilience and overall inflammation levels – a cool payoff for a cool practice!

- **Prioritize Sleep and Recovery:** Never underestimate the power of good sleep for your vagus nerve and immune system. During deep sleep, your body goes into full rest-and-digest mode – vagal activity dominates, heart rate drops, and your cells repair themselves. This nightly vagus activation is one reason consistent sleep is linked to stronger immunity. On the flip side, lack of sleep or poor-quality sleep is a known immune suppressant and inflammation booster. Have you ever noticed that after a few nights of bad sleep you might catch a cold or feel achy? It's no coincidence – sleep deprivation raises inflammatory cytokines and stresses your system. Make it a habit to get 7–9 hours of sleep per night and maintain a regular sleep schedule. Create a calming pre-bed routine (dim lights, no screens, maybe some light reading or meditation) to help engage your vagus nerve for better sleep. Additionally, incorporate moments of rest and downtime during the day. Short naps, leisurely walks, or even mindfulness breaks allow your vagus nerve to send out recovery signals. Remember, strengthening your vagus isn't only about active stimulation; it's also about avoiding chronic overdrive. By giving yourself permission to rest, you nurture a state of balance where healing can occur. Over time, these patterns of good sleep and rest will bolster both your vagal tone *and* your immune defenses – meaning you'll not only feel more refreshed, but you'll likely get sick less often and recover faster when you do.

By embracing these habits, you are essentially cultivating a "vagus lifestyle" – a way of living that constantly engages your body's natural healing power. Regular exercise pumps up anti-inflammatory signals, deep breathing and meditation turn down stress and tune up immunity, a bit of cold therapy challenges and strengthens your parasympathetic response, and quality sleep gives your system the recovery it craves. Individually, each of these habits can make a positive difference; together, they create a synergistic effect that can transform your health. You'll be reducing the chronic inflammation that silently contributes to aging and disease, and creating an internal environment where your body's natural healing processes can flourish. Best of all, these practices are simple and accessible – no fancy equipment or expensive programs required, just a commitment to self-care and consistency. As you integrate these vagus-friendly habits into daily life, you may notice you feel calmer, more energetic, and more resilient. That's the beauty of the vagus lifestyle: by strengthening this remarkable nerve, you're not just doing one thing – you're improving *everything* from your sleep to your mood to your immune system's ability to keep you healthy. In the journey to live longer, sleep better, and heal stronger, your vagus nerve might just be your best ally, and these daily habits are how you keep that ally in top shape.

By now, you've seen how the vagus nerve orchestrates an anti-inflammatory reflex that protects and heals us. It's like having a personal healing coach inside your body, ready to spring into action with the right cues. Strengthening your vagal tone through lifestyle not only helps keep inflammation in check, but also leaves you feeling more balanced and in charge of your well-being. In upcoming chapters, we'll continue to build on this knowledge – exploring more techniques and habits that leverage the vagus nerve to improve mental health, sleep, and overall vitality. But for now, give yourself credit: you're learning to speak the body's language of healing. Every deep breath, every evening walk, every good night's sleep – they're all messages that tell your vagus nerve, "Help is wanted here," and your body responds in kind with calm, repair, and strength. That is the essence of the vagus lifestyle, and it's a powerful path to a healthier, longer life.

The concept of the vagal inflammatory reflex and its ability to inhibit cytokine release was first identified by researchers like Dr. Kevin Tracey. Chronic inflammation's role in diseases (from arthritis to Alzheimer's) and the vagus nerve's balancing effect are well documented. Case studies and trials have shown vagus-oriented practices (e.g., meditation, yoga) reducing arthritis symptoms, and vagus nerve stimulators lowering inflammatory markers in patients. Experts in neuroimmunology explain that stress weakens immunity while vagus activation lowers stress and inflammation. Current medical research is actively exploring vagus nerve stimulation for conditions like rheumatoid arthritis, Crohn's disease, depression, and even long COVID, highlighting the serious scientific interest in the vagus nerve's healing potential. Practical habits such as exercise, which boosts vagal tone and lowers CRP, breathwork and cold exposure that activate vagus pathways, and sufficient sleep (to prevent inflammatory imbalance) are all supported by clinical research and are recommended for enhancing vagal tone and immunity. By combining these insights, we paint a comprehensive picture of how strengthening the vagus nerve through daily habits can keep inflammation in check and pave the way for better health and healing.

# Chapter 5

# Emotional Balance and the Brain – The Vagus Nerve's Impact on Mental Health

## The Mind-Body Link: Vagus Nerve as a Bridge Between Mental and Physical Health

The vagus nerve is a key structural link between our mind and body. Think of it as a two-way communication highway connecting your brain to your heart, lungs, gut, and more. Signals traveling along the vagus nerve don't just regulate your heartbeat or digestion – they also influence your mood and mental state. For example, stimulating the vagus can affect the release of neurotransmitters like serotonin and norepinephrine in brain regions tied to mood. In essence, what happens in your body (via the vagus nerve) can shape how you feel emotionally, and vice versa. This is why stress or anxiety often comes with physical sensations (racing heart, tense stomach) – and why calming the body can calm the mind. The vagus nerve serves as a bridge between mental and physical health, constantly sending signals back and forth to keep the two in balance.

One important concept here is *vagal tone*, which is a measure of how well your vagus nerve is functioning. High vagal tone generally means your vagus nerve is responsive and strong; low vagal tone means it's weaker or sluggish. Research shows a clear difference in emotional stability between high and low vagal tone. High vagal tone is associated with a calmer baseline and greater resilience to stress. People with higher vagal activity tend to recover faster from stress – their bodies more quickly activate the "rest and digest" response to put the brakes on the stress reaction. Physically, high vagal tone goes along with things like a lower resting heart rate and healthy digestion, but mentally it manifests as a sense of calm and ability to cope. On the other hand, low vagal tone is linked to anxiety, mood swings, and even a higher risk of depression. When vagal tone is low, the parasympathetic "braking" system isn't as effective, so the body stays in fight-or-flight mode longer and has a harder time settling down. Over time, this can leave a person feeling chronically on-edge, easily overwhelmed, and emotionally drained. Indeed, studies have found that low vagal tone often corresponds with heightened stress reactivity and difficulty regulating emotions.

In other words, when your vagus nerve is strong and responsive, you're more emotionally resilient – your body can effectively "put on the brakes" during stress, preventing those feelings of overwhelm. Instead of panic snowballing, a healthy vagus response helps slow your heart rate, relax your muscles, and stabilize your breathing. You might still feel stress, but you can ride the wave without being consumed by it. In contrast, if vagal tone is low, that internal brake doesn't work as well – so stress and negative emotions can spiral out of control more easily. This mind-body link explains why tending to your vagus nerve is also tending to your mental well-being. By improving vagal tone (through the kinds of habits we'll discuss), you're essentially strengthening your nervous system's ability to keep you calm, centered, and emotionally balanced.

It's fascinating to note that modern medicine is even leveraging this vagus-mental health connection: electronic vagus nerve stimulation (VNS) therapies have been shown to influence mood by sending signals into the brain. Researchers have observed that stimulating the vagus nerve can engage the same brain areas that depression affects and boost levels of mood-related brain chemicals. While those are high-tech treatments, the core lesson is the same – *our emotional state is deeply intertwined with our bodily state via the vagus nerve.* Cultivating a healthy vagal tone means your body and brain are better at working together to maintain a calm baseline. It's like having a resilient emotional buffer: you stay steadier during the day and bounce back faster when life pushes you off balance.

Case Study – Finding Calm and Joy Through Vagus-Focused Practices

To see this mind-body link in action, let's look at a real-life example. *A young woman in her 20s – we'll call her "M." for anonymity – had been struggling with depression and anxiety.* For M., daily life felt like walking on a tightrope. She woke each morning with a knot in her stomach and a racing heart, and the smallest setback could send her into a tailspin of worry. Some days, even an everyday challenge like an unexpected work deadline or a social invitation would trigger panic – her chest would tighten, thoughts would race, and she'd feel utterly overwhelmed by emotion. M. described it as "constantly living on the verge of fight-or-flight," and it was exhausting. She had trouble sleeping through the night and often felt emotionally drained by late afternoon, prone to mood swings and tears.

Traditional talk therapy and medication provided some help, but M. was searching for additional tools to regain a sense of calm and control in her life.

That's when she learned about techniques to strengthen the vagus nerve. A therapist suggested that by intentionally engaging her body's calming pathways (essentially, toning her vagus nerve), she might find some relief from the constant anxiety. Willing to try anything that could help her feel better, M. began incorporating a few simple vagus-focused practices into her daily routine. The first thing she tried was deep breathing exercises. Every morning and evening, she set aside 10 minutes to practice slow, diaphragmatic breathing – inhaling deeply into her belly for a count of 4, and exhaling slowly for a count of 6 or 8. At first, it was hard to sit still and focus on her breath (her mind would dart back to worries), but she stuck with it. After about a week, M. noticed something subtle: during her breathing practice she would actually feel her body softening. Her heart rate slowed and a sense of quiet calm would wash over her. It didn't solve all her problems overnight, but it gave her a glimpse of peace. In fact, she learned that this kind of deep, slow breathing was sending a signal through her vagus nerve telling her body it was safe to relax – essentially dialing down the stress response. This was empowering for M. because it was a tool she could use anytime, anywhere when anxiety flared up.

Encouraged by this, M. added mindfulness meditation to her routine as well. She started with just 5-10 minutes a day of sitting quietly, focusing on her breath or a simple mantra, and gently redirecting her thoughts when they wandered. Meditation was challenging at first (she joked that her brain felt like a web browser with 20 tabs open), but gradually she found it became easier to drop into a calm, present state. On the days she meditated, she noticed she felt a bit less reactive and more grounded. Little inconveniences – like a traffic jam or a rude email – didn't send her into panic as often. It was as if that "tight spring" inside her was loosening. Physiologically, what M. was doing with meditation was similar to the breathing exercises: activating her parasympathetic nervous system through the vagus nerve. Over time, those daily moments of calm started to carry over into the rest of her day.

The most transformative change, however, came when M. found a way to bring *joy* and social connection back into her life. On a friend's encouragement, she joined a local community singing group that met once a week. M. had loved singing in high school but had fallen out of the habit during her difficult times. The group turned out to be a lighthearted choir that met to sing upbeat, uplifting songs just for fun – no pressure to perform perfectly. The first evening she went, M. was shy and almost backed out at the door. But as the group warmed up with a silly humming exercise and then launched into a familiar song, she found herself smiling for the first time in a long time. By the end of that session, she was laughing and harmonizing with people she had just met. She walked home feeling almost euphoric. More importantly, she noticed that on the days following choir practice, her mood was noticeably brighter and her anxiety lower. It wasn't just the distraction – there seemed to be a lingering physiological calm that stayed with her.

In hindsight, several things were happening during those singing sessions. Singing – especially in a group – is a natural vagus nerve stimulator. The act of singing involves deep, controlled breaths and prolonged exhalation (when phrasing through lyrics), which activates the vagus nerve similarly to formal breathing exercises. Even humming or chanting causes vibrations in the throat that directly stimulate branches of the vagus nerve. M. didn't know the science at first, but she definitely felt the effects: her body would be in a relaxed, happy state after each session. On top of that, the social connection of singing with others in unison gave her a powerful sense of safety and belonging. She later learned that feeling socially connected signals the vagus nerve that you're safe, which further boosts its calming activity. In the choir, M. felt welcomed and supported – a stark contrast to the isolation she felt when her depression was at its worst. It makes sense that this warmth and camaraderie helped "flip the switch" in her nervous system from stress to rest. (There's a reason we often feel calm and happy after a night of laughter with friends; positive social engagement is like a natural tonic for the vagus nerve.)

Emboldened by her progress, M. also tried a laughter yoga class that she heard about through the community center. She admitted it felt extremely silly at first – a group of adults making intentional giggles and guffaws for no reason! But the silliness itself was infectious. Before she knew it, real laughter was bubbling up. In those moments of hearty, tear-streaming laughter, M. could physically feel tension releasing from her body. Later that night, she slept deeper than she had in months. It turns out that deep belly laughter can literally massage your organs and stimulate vagal activity, triggering a wave of relaxation. As one clinician put it, *when we laugh, cortisol levels drop and laughter "helps tone your vagus nerve," a key player in stress reduction.* M. certainly found that to be true – a good laugh became one of her favorite medicines. Even on tough days, if she could watch a 10-minute clip of a comedy show or recall a funny memory to prompt some laughter, it would shift her mood and soothe her frazzled nerves.

After a couple of months of consistently practicing these vagus-friendly habits, M.'s transformation was remarkable. She went from living in a near-constant state of anxiety and gloom to feeling *steady* and even optimistic. She still had normal ups and downs, of course, but the pendulum didn't swing so wildly anymore. Importantly, when stress did come (and life being life, it did), she found she could handle it without spiraling. For instance, one afternoon her boss assigned a major project with a tight deadline – something that would have definitely triggered a panic attack in the past. M. felt a flash of nerves, but she instinctively paused, took a few slow, deep breaths, and then started tackling the work methodically. "It was like I finally found the brake pedal for my anxiety," she later explained. Strengthening her vagal tone through breathing, meditation, singing, and laughter had given her body the ability to put on the brakes during stress, preventing that feeling of being overwhelmed. Instead of her heart racing out of control and her mind flooding with doom, she experienced a sense of *"I've got this, I can cope."* This newfound resilience opened the door for more positive experiences – she began socializing more, pursuing hobbies again, and even noted improvements in her sleep and energy levels. M.'s story illustrates in personal terms what science has been discovering: when you actively tone your vagus nerve, you nurture your emotional balance. By engaging in simple daily practices, she essentially taught her body how to feel safe again, and her mind was able to blossom in that safety. Less anxiety, more joy – that is the vagus lifestyle in action.

## The Polyvagal Perspective: Why Feeling Safe Calms Your Mind (Expert Insight)

To delve deeper into *why* the vagus nerve has such an impact on mental health, it helps to understand the Polyvagal Theory, developed by neuroscientist Dr. Stephen Porges. Polyvagal Theory gives us a framework for understanding how our sense of safety (or danger) switches different "paths" in our nervous system, with the vagus nerve playing a central role. In simple terms, Porges's work suggests that the vagus nerve isn't just one uniform nerve – it actually has multiple branches that evolved over time, and these support our ability to connect socially and regulate our emotions. One branch (often called the ventral vagal pathway) is the newer, "social" vagus; when this pathway is active, we feel safe, calm, and socially engaged. Another branch is the older vagal circuit (the dorsal vagal pathway), which comes into play in situations of extreme threat – it can trigger a shutdown or freeze response. Between these vagal systems and our sympathetic "fight-or-flight" system, our body has a sort of ladder of responses to the world. Let's break it down:

- **Safe and Social State (Ventral Vagal Activation):** When your brain perceives that you are safe, the ventral vagal branch is in charge. In this state, your heart rate is steady and slow, you can relax, digest, and even connect with others. You feel grounded and open. Porges explains that in safe contexts, when our mammalian vagal circuits are active, our nervous system functions optimally – supporting health, digestion, and social communication. *"In 'safe' contexts, when our mammalian vagal circuits are active, the function of our nervous system is optimized to support processes related to health, growth, and restoration as well as connectedness and intimacy,"* Dr. Porges notes. This is the state where you might describe yourself as "at ease" or "content." You're not just mentally calm; your whole body is in a restorative mode thanks to the vagus nerve steadily signaling safety. In safe mode, we naturally seek out social interaction – we can make eye contact, listen, and converse, all of which further reinforces the feeling of safety. (Interestingly, the ventral vagal pathways link to the muscles of the face and voice, which is why, for example, a genuine warm smile or a soothing tone of voice can immediately put someone at ease – our bodies are literally wired to use these social signals to calm each other.)

- **Fight-or-Flight State (Sympathetic Activation, Ventral Vagal Off-Line):** Now, if something in our environment is perceived as dangerous or threatening, our brain shifts gears. It essentially "turns off" that social-calm vagal circuit for a while and activates the sympathetic nervous system – the classic fight-or-flight response. You've likely felt this: it's when your heart starts pounding, breathing quickens, and muscles tense up ready to run or fight. Porges describes this shift, saying that when we no longer feel safe, the ventral vagal system goes off-line and we become more defensive and disconnected. In this mode, our body is focused on pure survival – you might feel anxious, angry, or just on high alert. Our higher social brain functions (like logical reasoning or empathy) get dialed down because all systems are directed toward dealing with the threat. As Dr. Porges put it, we *"fall prey to sympathetic nervous system stress – the fight or flight reflex – which shuts down much of our higher social brain"*. This is why when you're highly anxious or panicked, it's very hard to socialize or think clearly; your biology is in survival mode, not social mode. Notably, the vagus nerve is still involved here, but instead of actively calming things, it's sort of "releasing the brakes" to allow your heart rate and stress response to rev up in defense. (In Polyvagal terms, the ventral vagal brake is disengaged to let the heart pump faster for fight/flight.)

- **Shutdown or Freeze State (Dorsal Vagal Activation):** There's a third state that happens if the perceived threat is extreme and fight-or-flight doesn't resolve it. This is the freeze or collapse response, governed by the older dorsal branch of the vagus nerve. It's like the body's last resort: playing dead, numbing out, or conserving energy by shutting down. You might have experienced a mild version of this as that feeling of being emotionally overwhelmed to the point of emptiness or fatigue (some people describe dissociating or "checking out" under intense stress). Porges notes that in life-threatening situations, our bodies may trigger this ancient vagal circuit – essentially causing fainting, shutting down, or immobilization. It's not a conscious decision; it's an automatic "off switch" when the nervous system is maxed out. In everyday mental health terms, this could correspond to episodes of dissociation, extreme fatigue during depression, or the sense of "numbing" in trauma. It's the polar opposite of social engagement – it's the body's way of escaping by going inward and quiet. While this state can be protective in truly dangerous situations, staying in a shutdown mode for too long isn't healthy for us either.

What Polyvagal Theory highlights is that feeling safe is critical for our emotional wellness. Our vagus nerve is constantly sensing the world (through what Porges calls "neuroception") and asking, *"Am I safe right now, or am I in danger?"* If we feel safe – say, relaxed at home with a good friend – our vagal "social" system comes online and keeps us calm and connected. But if we sense threat – even something like the stress of a loud, chaotic environment or the emotional threat of conflict – our body might shift into fight/flight or freeze, disrupting that calm state. This is happening beneath our conscious awareness. As one description puts it, *the vagus nerve's duty is to orchestrate bodily responses to keep you safe or warn you about danger before you even think about it. The brain constantly scans for danger cues (triggering high alert to fight or flee, or shutting down if it's overwhelming), and it also scans for cues of safety, which allow you to relax enough to socially engage with others.*

Knowing this, we can better understand why certain activities naturally soothe our nerves. Activities that send "cues of safety" will activate the ventral vagal pathway and calm us down. For example, slow, deep breathing is a cue of safety – it's something your body only does when it feels safe (think about it: if you were in immediate danger, you wouldn't be taking slow breaths, you'd be hyperventilating). So deliberately breathing slowly is like telling your brain, "It's okay, you can relax," and your vagus nerve responds by pumping the brakes on anxiety. Similarly, positive social interactions – like a warm face-to-face conversation, gentle eye contact, or a caring hug – reassure your nervous system that you're among allies, not enemies. That triggers the vagus nerve to keep you in that social-and-safe mode. It's the reason why your *body* relaxes when a friend smiles and says "I'm happy to see you" – your vagus nerve is reading that cue and maintaining your calm state. On the flip side, if you encounter angry yelling or a threatening glare, your body might tense up before you even mentally process what's happening; that's the vagus and its partner nerves sensing danger and preparing you.

To lend some expert credibility to this, Dr. Porges's insights again are useful. He emphasizes that our need to feel safe is a primal drive and that social connectivity is actually a built-in vagal calming system. When you feel securely connected – whether it's bonding with a loved one or even bonding with a pet – you activate that ventral vagal state of calm and trust. The Polyvagal perspective essentially says that by finding ways to make our body feel safe, we can stabilize our emotions. It provides a scientific explanation for why things like breathing exercises, meditation, and positive socializing (the same practices M. used in the case study) have such a powerful effect on mental health. They are all ways of feeding safety cues into our nervous system, thereby engaging the vagus nerve's calming influence. An experienced therapist might put it this way: *you can't talk someone out of anxiety if their body is stuck in fight-or-flight; you have to signal to their body that it's safe first.* The vagus nerve is the channel for that signal.

The takeaway from the Polyvagal Theory is a reassuring one. It tells us that our bodies have an inherent system for emotional regulation – a kind of internal emotional thermostat – rooted in the vagus nerve. When we learn how to work *with* that system (through breathing, mindful awareness of safety, etc.), we gain a powerful tool for mental health. We essentially become active participants in calming our own nervous system. Feeling safe, socially connected, and grounded isn't just a vague notion; it's a physiological state triggered by the vagus nerve. And with some practice, we can learn to enter that state more readily, strengthening our "vagal tone" just like exercising a muscle.

## Mood-Boosting Vagus Exercises: Practical Techniques for Emotional Well-Being

By now it's clear that engaging the vagus nerve can foster emotional balance – so how can you do that in daily life? This section offers a set of fun, simple practices to improve your vagal tone and uplift your mood. The best part is that these techniques are enjoyable *and* they have a real physiological impact. Essentially, they stimulate your parasympathetic nervous system (the calming "rest and digest" side) via the vagus nerve, strengthening your body's natural relaxation response over time. Consider incorporating these exercises into your week – even a few minutes can make a difference. Not only will you likely feel comforted or energized by these activities, but you'll also be literally training your body to be more resilient and happy through the "vagus brain-body" connection.

- **Sing or Hum Your Favorite Tune:** Whether you belt out a song in the shower, hum along to the radio, or join a local choir, using your voice can directly stimulate your vagus nerve. The vibrations from humming and the regulated breath control from singing are a one-two punch for vagal activation. In fact, therapists note that making sounds – humming, singing, even gargling – massages muscles in the throat connected to the vagus nerve and increases something called heart rate variability, a marker of healthy vagal tone. If you've ever noticed how singing a song can lift your spirits, there's science behind that feeling! Singing triggers the release of endorphins and often dopamine (because it's joyful), but concurrently it's activating your vagus nerve which promotes calm. It's a wonderful mix of energizing and soothing. Don't worry, you don't have to be *good* at singing – this is purely for you. Try incorporating a "humming break" in your day: spend a minute or two humming a calming melody (the slower and more melodious, the better for relaxation). You might feel a pleasant vibration in your chest and throat; that's a good sign your vagus nerve is being stimulated. Over time, this practice can help lower stress and improve your overall mood. Bonus points if you do it with others (like singing together with friends or in a group), because the social aspect can further amplify the positive effects. Singing in unison has even been studied in research – it tends to synchronize heart rates and promote social bonding, giving you a double dose of vagal tone and happiness.

- **Laugh It Out (Seriously!):** Laughter is truly "internal jogging." Genuine laughter exercises your diaphragm, gets your lungs pumping, and triggers a cascade of positive physical effects – many of which involve the vagus nerve. A good hearty laugh actually stimulates the vagus nerve, sending signals that reduce stress hormone levels. For example, studies have shown that during laughter, levels of cortisol (a primary stress hormone) drop, while vagal activity goes up. Think about the last time you had a big belly laugh – you probably felt a release of tension and a sense of relief afterward. That's the vagus nerve at work, calming your system. To harness this, make laughter a deliberate practice. You might try laughter yoga (classes or videos where you engage in guided laughing exercises – it sounds odd but can be incredibly effective and fun), or simply curate a list of go-to comedies, funny YouTube clips, or humorous podcasts that crack you up. Even spending time with a friend who gives you the giggles is wonderful "vagus therapy." The key is deep, spontaneous laughter – the kind that makes you exhale forcefully and maybe even wipes tears from your eyes. Those deep exhalations and diaphragmatic movements during laughter are essentially giving your internal organs a gentle massage and activating vagal nerve fibers. One healthcare article succinctly noted, "having a good laugh lifts your mood, boosts your immune system and stimulates the vagus nerve". So don't dismiss laughter as trivial – it's physiologically powerful. Aim to laugh *with gusto* each day, even if it means laughing at your own silliness. It will not only brighten your mood but also strengthen your body's relaxation response.

- **Practice Gratitude and Loving-Kindness:** Cultivating positive emotions like gratitude, compassion, and love can have a surprisingly strong impact on your vagus nerve. Emotional practices such as gratitude journaling or loving-kindness meditation (also known as Metta meditation, where you silently send good wishes to yourself and others) do more than just "feel nice" – they can shift your body into a state of safety and social connection, boosting vagal tone. Research has demonstrated a fascinating upward spiral: when people regularly generated positive feelings (through practices like loving-kindness meditation), they not only felt more socially connected, but their vagal tone measurably increased over time. In one study, those who did a brief loving-kindness meditation each day showed improvements in their heart rate variability (a proxy for vagus nerve activity) and reported greater positive emotions and social bonds compared to those who didn't. The mechanism seems to be that positive social emotions signal to your nervous system that you're in a supportive, safe environment – essentially turning "on" the ventral vagal system we discussed. Even simple acts of kindness or moments of heartfelt gratitude can send these signals. For example, reflecting each night on a few things you're grateful for can evoke feelings of contentment and safety. An article from

Massachusetts General Hospital put it plainly: activities like *expressing gratitude, doing acts of kindness, and fostering social connection all support healthy vagus nerve function.* You can practice this in many forms: try writing a thank-you note to someone who made a difference in your life, spend a few minutes in the morning thinking of people you love and silently wishing them well, or incorporate a short loving-kindness meditation in your week. Not only do these practices shift your mindset toward the positive, but physiologically they increase parasympathetic (vagal) activity, which over time can lower stress levels and even improve things like heart health. It's a beautiful example of how tending to the spirit (kindness, love, gratitude) also tends to the body.

As you integrate these mood-boosting vagus exercises into your life, remember that consistency is more impactful than intensity. Small daily habits – a song here, a laugh there, a moment of gratitude at day's end – can compound into a significant improvement in your baseline mood and stress resilience. They are enjoyable rituals that also happen to be "workouts" for your vagus nerve, strengthening your body's natural healing and calming powers. Make it fun: perhaps have a weekly game night or comedy night with friends (social connection + laughter = vagus goldmine), or a morning routine that includes a favorite song to hum and a few grateful breaths. Over time, these practices help build a *resilient, happy mind* by leveraging the vagus nerve's profound influence on our emotional life. Living the "vagus lifestyle" means recognizing that by caring for this mind-body nexus, we give ourselves the gift of emotional balance and a more joyful, healthier life. With a strong vagus nerve on your side, you're not at the mercy of stress – you have inner brakes you can tap, and pathways of calm you can activate, whenever you need them. Enjoy the process of experimenting with these techniques, and take heart in the knowledge that each deep breath, each song, each shared laugh, and each kind thought is bringing your mind and body into greater harmony. Your emotional well-being is literally within you – in that wandering vagus nerve – and by nurturing it, you are truly tending to both body *and* mind in the most natural way.

# Chapter 6

# Gut Feelings – Nutrition, Digestion, and the Vagus Nerve

## The Gut-Brain Axis Explained

Have you ever felt "butterflies" in your stomach when anxious, or a gut instinct about something? It turns out these gut feelings are rooted in a real biological dialogue between your digestive system and your brain. This communication superhighway is often called the gut-brain axis, and at its center is the vagus nerve – a cranial nerve so extensive and influential that it's nicknamed the "wandering nerve." The vagus nerve is essentially the main line connecting your brain to your intestinal tract. Think of it as a two-way phone line: it carries commands from the brain to the gut, and a wealth of sensory information from the gut back up to the brain. In fact, roughly 80% of the vagus nerve's fibers are afferent, meaning they send information upward from our organs (especially the digestive tract) to the brain. This means our gut health can send powerful signals that shape our mood and energy levels, not just the other way around. It's no wonder we say we "feel" things in our gut – the gut is literally in constant conversation with the brain about how we're doing.

When you sit down to a meal, your vagus nerve orchestrates digestion. Under the parasympathetic "rest and digest" mode, the vagus tells your stomach to release acid and your pancreas to secrete digestive enzymes, while also coordinating the muscular waves (motility) that move food along your intestines. This nerve pathway helps ensure that when you eat, your body is ready to break down food and absorb nutrients efficiently. It even plays a role in signaling satiety – as your stomach stretches with food, vagal sensors help relay fullness signals to your brain, telling you when you've had enough. (Ever notice how eating slowly gives you time to realize you're full? That's your vagus nerve at work.) Because the vagus has fingers on the dial of so many digestive functions, if its tone or activity is low, things can go awry. Impaired vagus function can lead to issues like acid reflux, delayed stomach emptying, or even irritable bowel syndrome (IBS). On the flip side, a healthy, active vagus nerve tends to promote smooth digestion and regularity.

A remarkable fact is that the information flow on the gut-brain axis is mostly from gut to brain – the vagus nerve is constantly reporting on the state of affairs in your gastrointestinal tract. Is there enough nutrient intake? Are there any toxins detected? How are the gut microbes doing? About four-fifths of the vagal fibers are carrying these sensory updates upward, influencing brain regions involved in emotion, stress response, and even memory. Because of this, scientists have come to appreciate that our gut health can directly influence our mental state. A balanced, well-functioning gut can send "all is well" signals that promote a stable mood and good energy. Conversely, an upset or inflamed gut can sound the alarm through the vagus nerve, potentially contributing to feelings of anxiety, low energy, or brain fog. As the Cleveland Clinic notes, the crosstalk between gut and brain can affect everything from hunger and satiety to mood and stress levels. This sets the stage for a powerful idea: *what* we eat and *how* we eat can affect vagal tone (the activity of the vagus nerve), and vagal tone in turn can affect our digestion and overall well-being. In short, caring for your gut means caring for your mind, and the vagus nerve is the friendly mediator in between.

To put it simply, the gut-brain axis is the reason why a nervous thought can cause an upset stomach, or why a meal eaten in a calm, happy environment just seems to "sit" better. Understanding this connection gives us a new appreciation for nutrition and digestion: it's not just about calories or nutrients, it's about signaling. Every meal is an opportunity to send good signals through the vagus nerve – signals of satiety, safety, and satisfaction – that resonate through both body and brain. And as we'll explore, by optimizing those signals through smart eating habits, we can improve our vagal tone, aiding digestion, boosting mood, and even supporting the body's natural healing responses.

## Case Study – Healing the Gut

Let's bring this mind-gut connection to life with a real-world example. Meet Elena, a 38-year-old graphic designer with a lifelong "sensitive stomach." Elena suffers from Irritable Bowel Syndrome (IBS) – her belly would bloat painfully on random days, and stress only made it worse. Rushing to meet deadlines at work, she often ate lunch at her desk, barely chewing as she worried about emails. It was a recipe for digestive disaster. Sure enough, on stressful days her intestines seemed tied in knots. Doctors told Elena that IBS is often exacerbated by stress (the brain-gut axis at work), and she noticed the pattern too – whenever she felt anxious or overworked, her gut symptoms flared. Stress triggers the "fight or flight" response, which can interfere with digestion by slowing down gut motility and even changing how the brain perceives pain signals from the gut. Elena's experience fit that mold exactly: stress was revving up her sympathetic nerves and putting the brakes on her vagus nerve, leading to cramping, irregularity, and discomfort.

Desperate for relief, Elena decided to address her problem from both ends – mind and body. She consulted a holistic gastroenterologist who emphasized that calming her nervous system was just as important as changing her diet. The doctor explained that when we activate the vagus nerve, we engage the "rest and digest" response, which can help untangle that knotted-up feeling in the gut. Elena started a new routine: before each meal, she'd do a short breathing exercise to stimulate her vagus nerve and enter a relaxed state. She would sit down, close her eyes for a minute, and take slow, deep breaths from her diaphragm. At first she felt a bit silly, but it soon became her favorite ritual. Indeed, just taking slow, deep breaths triggers a relaxation response in the body, switching off fight-or-flight and allowing digestion to proceed smoothly. This simple practice essentially told her vagus nerve, "It's okay to digest now." Elena learned that this wasn't fluff – breathing deeply signals the vagus nerve to lower heart rate and boost gut motility, essentially giving her body permission to direct resources to digestion instead of to stress responses.

Along with breathing and a more mindful, unrushed approach to meals, Elena also revamped *what* she was eating. She cut down on the ultra-processed convenience foods she used to grab when busy, and instead tried to include more gut-friendly foods her doctor recommended. She added a daily probiotic yogurt or kefir in the mornings, started having a colorful salad with mixed vegetables (for fiber) at lunch, and incorporated fermented foods like kimchi or sauerkraut with dinner a few times a week. These foods are rich in beneficial bacteria and fibers that support a healthy gut microbiome. Why does that matter? Because a healthy gut microbiome means a healthier gut-brain axis – those microbes produce neurotransmitters and reduce inflammation, sending better signals up the vagus nerve. Elena also made sure to include sources of omega-3 fatty acids (like salmon and walnuts) a couple times a week after learning they can help calm inflammation in the gut. And importantly, she didn't just change *what* she ate; she changed *how* she ate. Gone were the days of scarfing a sandwich in 5 minutes; now, she made a point to sit down for 20–30 minutes, chew thoroughly, and actually savor her food. She even practiced a bit of gratitude before meals, thinking of something positive or the farmers who grew her food – anything to cultivate positive feelings and signal safety to her body. It turns out expressing gratitude and eating with awareness can lower stress hormones and prepare your body to digest more effectively. Elena's entire mealtime environment transformed from a drive-by fueling to a mini oasis of calm.

The results were subtle at first. The first week, she still had some bloating, but she noticed she burped less and didn't feel as painfully stuffed after eating. After a month of consistency, Elena's digestion had dramatically calmed. She was having regular bowel movements every morning, almost like clockwork. The bloating that used to sabotage her afternoons became a rarity. And if stressors popped up – a tough client call or a traffic jam – she found that a few deep belly breaths could prevent those stress butterflies from lodging in her gut. Over a few months, Elena's IBS flares became infrequent and much milder. She recalls one day realizing, "Hey, I haven't had a bad stomach day in weeks!" Her abdominal pain diminished, and so did her anxiety around food. By engaging the vagus nerve through relaxation techniques and feeding her body nutritious, gut-soothing foods, she had essentially broken the vicious cycle of stress and poor digestion that had plagued her. This case illustrates a powerful lesson: when we calm the nervous system and "feed the gut right," the gut often heals – and it sends signals of relief and balance back to the brain. Elena not only felt physically better but also more energetic and upbeat, as if lifting the burden of digestive woes lifted her mood as well.

Now, Elena's story is just one example, but it reflects a common truth for many with stress-related digestive issues. IBS, in particular, is known to be aggravated by stress and associated with a low vagal tone (research shows many IBS patients have reduced vagus nerve activity). By consciously activating her vagus nerve (with breathing and mindfulness) and improving her gut health (with diet), Elena addressed both sides of the gut-brain axis. The improvements she experienced – less bloating, better regularity, reduced gut pain – are echoed by research that finds stress reduction and mindful eating can relieve IBS symptoms. This "healing the gut from inside and out" approach may sound simple, but it's profoundly effective. It's empowering to realize that by changing daily habits, we hold a key to influencing this deep, mind-body connection.

Elena's journey shows that our brains and bellies can work in harmony when given the right support, leading to calmer digestion, a calmer mind, and a happier daily life.

## Expert Guidance on Food & Mood

With so much buzz around the vagus nerve and gut health, it's worth getting some clear, science-backed advice on how diet and vagal tone work together. For this, let's turn to what the experts say – nutritionists and gastroenterologists who bridge the gap between what we eat and how we feel. One key piece of guidance that comes up again and again is: *take care of your gut microbiome*. According to nutritional psychiatrists like Dr. Uma Naidoo of Harvard, a diverse and balanced gut microbiome (the community of bacteria in your intestines) is essential for mental well-being, and diet is the fastest way to shape it. Eating more fiber and fermented foods is often recommended to support those good gut bugs. Fiber (found in fruits, vegetables, whole grains, legumes) is like a daily buffet for beneficial bacteria – when bacteria ferment fiber, they produce short-chain fatty acids that reduce inflammation and even influence brain function. Fermented foods (like yogurt, kefir, kimchi, sauerkraut) directly add friendly microbes and have been shown to benefit the gut-brain axis. As Dr. Naidoo notes, fermented foods can help maintain a healthy gut lining and even alter brain activity in positive ways. And a gut that's well-fed and flourishing communicates more optimistically with the brain via the vagus nerve. So, the expert consensus is to nourish your microbiome with whole, natural foods rather than processed ones.

Experts also caution against the idea that you can simply pop a pill to "hack" the vagus nerve. You might have heard that certain supplements – say omega-3 fish oil or probiotic capsules – can *stimulate* vagus nerve activity. This is a popular talking point on wellness blogs, but what do researchers say? At present, there isn't evidence that any supplement directly boosts vagal tone or nerve signals. For example, omega-3 fatty acids are fantastic for overall health and reducing inflammation, and probiotics can support a healthy gut environment, but no study has shown that taking these leads to a measurable change in your vagus nerve's function. This doesn't mean they're useless – far from it. It just means their benefits (heart health, lower inflammation, better immunity, etc.) likely *indirectly* help the gut-brain axis rather than working like a magic on/off switch for the vagus. A gastroenterologist might say: focus on the big picture of an anti-inflammatory diet and stress management, and be wary of quick fixes claiming to "reset" your vagus nerve overnight.

So, what practical science-based tips do the experts agree on? Interestingly, one of the most effective "vagus nerve boosters" isn't a product at all – it's the way you slow down and eat your meals. Slow, mindful eating is a simple but profound habit. When you eat slowly and chew well, you activate the vagus nerve's role in sensing food and signaling satiety (fullness) in a timely manner, which can prevent overeating and improve digestion. In a hurried, distracted meal, you might shovel food in faster than your gut can say "Enough!", but in a relaxed meal, the vagus nerve has time to relay those fullness signals so you naturally feel satisfied with the right amount of food. Mindful eating also engages more of your senses and encourages the parasympathetic response, meaning your body is in "digest mode" rather than stress mode. As one wellness coach put it, *digestion begins in the mind.* Taking a moment of gratitude or simply appreciating the aroma and taste of your food can shift you into a calmer state. Clinical experts agree that thorough chewing and savoring your food can improve nutrient absorption and reduce digestive discomfort. It's a bit like giving your stomach a head start – chewing triggers saliva and digestive enzymes, and a calm mindset triggers the vagus nerve to start the digestive engines smoothly.

We also reached out to Dr. Anil Gupta, a gastroenterologist with a special interest in the gut-brain connection, for his perspective. He emphasized balance and consistency over fads. "There's a lot of hype out there," Dr. Gupta told us. "People ask if they should take this supplement to stimulate their vagus nerve or that superfood to cure their anxiety. The truth is, supporting your vagus nerve health is *not* about one exotic hack – it's about your daily habits." He advises his patients to adopt a whole-foods diet rich in vegetables, fruits, whole grains, lean proteins, and healthy fats, which naturally provides the fiber, vitamins, and minerals that both the gut and nervous system thrive on. "Your gut bacteria communicate with your brain through the vagus nerve," he explains, "so feed the bacteria well. They love fiber, they love fermented foods. Give them those, and they'll produce nutrients and neurotransmitters that keep your gut lining strong and your mood steady." On the other hand, he notes that diets high in refined sugars and processed foods tend to promote inflammation and disrupt the gut microbiome, which can send negative signals through the vagus nerve. It's telling that researchers say we should "fix the food first" before relying on pills – meaning clean up the diet to reduce gut inflammation and dysbiosis (microbial imbalance) as a foundational step. Dr. Gupta also chuckled about some trends: "I've had patients ask if *gargling* or *coffee enemas* will stimulate the vagus nerve. I tell them: maybe, but probably not as much as a good yoga class or a daily walk in nature." His point is that general wellness practices – stress reduction, good sleep, moderate exercise – are vagus-friendly because they tone your parasympathetic system.

Crucially, our experts underscore that diet and vagal tone go hand in hand with stress management. You can eat all the kale and kimchi in the world, but if you're eating it in a frantic state, your vagus nerve (and digestion) won't reap the full benefits. Thus, integrating mindfulness, enjoyable social connection at meals, and not eating on the run are part of the prescription. In summary, the expert guidance can be boiled down to this: *nourish the gut-brain axis with wholesome food and calming daily practices.* Avoid the temptation of extreme diets or miracle supplements for vagus nerve health. Instead, embrace simple habits like eating slowly, including gut-friendly foods, and taking moments of relaxation. These create the optimal conditions for your vagus nerve to do its job – keeping your digestion humming along and your brain-gut signals in happy balance.

## Nourish Your Vagus – Practical Tips

By now, you can see that supporting your vagus nerve is less about doing one big thing and more about small daily habits. The good news is many of these habits are pleasant and easy to integrate into your routine. Here is a menu of actionable tips to nourish your vagus nerve through nutrition and lifestyle:

- **Practice a "Gratitude Pause" Before Meals:** Before you dig in, take a brief pause. Close your eyes, take a few deep breaths, and acknowledge something you're grateful for – perhaps gratitude for the food, the people you're eating with, or simply a calm moment in the day. This simple ritual triggers a calm, parasympathetic state that primes your body for digestion. Deep breathing and positive thoughts lower stress hormones like cortisol, effectively telling your vagus nerve it's safe to enter "rest and digest" mode. You might be surprised how this enhances not only your digestion (food tends to sit better) but also your enjoyment of the meal.

- **Eat Mindfully – Slow Down and Chew:** In our fast-paced world, mindful eating is a game changer for vagus nerve health. Try to chew each bite thoroughly (aim for 20–30 chews) and truly taste your food. Eating slowly and without distraction (putting aside phones or screens) allows your gut-brain axis to synchronize. Remember, it takes a little time for your stomach's stretch receptors and gut hormones to signal your brain that you're getting full. When you eat slowly, you give the vagus nerve time to send those fullness and satisfaction signals, preventing overeating and discomfort. This practice also improves digestion – chewing well starts digestion in the mouth and leads to better nutrient absorption, with less chance of bloating. Make meals a sensory experience: notice the flavors, textures, and aromas. This not only makes eating more enjoyable, it also keeps you in a relaxed state that optimizes vagal activity and even mood.

- **Include Omega-3 Rich Foods:** Instead of thinking in terms of supplements, think in terms of foods. Omega-3 fatty acids, famous for their anti-inflammatory benefits, support overall brain and heart health *and* help maintain a healthy gut environment. Fatty fish like salmon, mackerel, and sardines are top sources of omega-3s, as are flaxseeds, chia seeds, and walnuts. By reducing inflammation, these foods create a more hospitable environment for your vagus nerve and gut. (Chronic inflammation can interfere with vagus nerve signaling, so keeping inflammation in check is key.) While fish oil capsules alone might not directly spike your vagal tone, eating omega-3 rich foods is definitely associated with lower inflammation and a healthier nervous system, which indirectly benefits vagus function. Try a couple of fish meals per week or sprinkle ground flax on your oatmeal – small additions can have big impacts over time.

- **Feed Your Gut with Probiotics and Prebiotics: Probiotic foods** – those containing live beneficial bacteria – can help repopulate your gut with good microbes. Yogurt (with live cultures), kefir, kombucha, miso, kimchi, and sauerkraut are great choices. For example, having a serving of unsweetened yogurt or kefir daily can introduce strains of bacteria that support your intestinal health. Meanwhile, prebiotic foods (the fiber that feeds those microbes) are just as important. Foods like garlic, onions, asparagus, bananas, and oats contain fibers that your gut bacteria ferment into nutrients that soothe and communicate with the gut lining. Together, probiotic and prebiotic foods help foster a robust microbiome, which in turn can positively influence your brain via vagus nerve signaling. Think of it this way: a diverse garden of microbes in your gut produces lots of helpful compounds (including some neurotransmitters), essentially giving your vagus nerve *happy news* to report to your brain. Aim to include some fermented food or drink each day, and load up on fiber-rich plant foods to keep your microscopic friends well-fed.

- **Cut Down on Highly Processed, Inflammatory Foods:** Our modern diet is flooded with ultra-processed items (sugary snacks, fast foods, processed meats, sodas) that can wreak havoc on the gut-brain axis. These foods often lead to inflammation in the gut and can disrupt the delicate balance of your microbiome. Inflammatory signals from the gut can overload the vagus nerve with distress messages. To keep your vagus nerve "tone" positive, minimize foods high in refined sugars, artificial additives, and unhealthy fats. Instead, choose whole foods as close to their natural form as possible. Research suggests that diets high in processed foods correlate with higher rates of mood issues and gut problems. Meanwhile, diets full of whole foods (like the Mediterranean diet) are linked to better mood and lower inflammation. As one guideline, when shopping, check labels – the fewer weird additives, the better. "Fix the food first" is sage advice. By avoiding the junk that aggravates your gut, you allow your microbiome and vagus nerve to function optimally, without constantly mounting an inflammatory defense. You'll likely notice the difference in how you feel: more energy, more mental clarity, and a happier gut after meals.

- **Stay Hydrated: Proper hydration is essential for healthy digestion** and vagus nerve function. Water helps break down food, absorb nutrients, and keeps the intestinal environment smooth and supple. Ever get constipated when you're dehydrated? That's a sign of how crucial water is for gut motility. Aim to drink plenty of fluids (mostly water) throughout the day. Hydration supports the volume of blood and lymph that carry nutrients to your nerves (including the vagus) and ensures that digestion moves along without trouble. A well-hydrated gut is less likely to be irritated, and thus less likely to send distress signals. In fact, staying hydrated aids nutrient absorption and overall gut function, creating conditions for the vagus nerve to relay *good* news to the brain. A simple habit is to drink a glass of water about 30 minutes before a meal – this can aid digestion, and you'll be less likely to confuse thirst with hunger. Also, remember that many fruits and veggies contribute fluids too, so a juicy apple or cucumber contributes to hydration while feeding your gut fiber.

- **Get Your Magnesium (Leafy Greens and More):** Magnesium is a mineral that deserves a shout-out when it comes to the nervous system. It's often nicknamed "nature's relaxant" because of its calming effect on nerves. Magnesium helps regulate neurotransmitters and assists in proper nerve signal transmission. In terms of the vagus nerve, magnesium's calming influence can indirectly support healthy vagal tone by reducing excessive firing of stress pathways. It's also involved in the production of acetylcholine, the main neurotransmitter used by the vagus nerve to communicate with organs. Sufficient magnesium helps ensure that when your vagus nerve sends a "relax and digest" signal, the message gets through loud and clear. To get magnesium through food, include leafy green vegetables (spinach, kale, Swiss chard), nuts and seeds (almonds, pumpkin seeds), legumes, and whole grains in your diet. For example, a cup of cooked spinach or a handful of almonds packs a good magnesium punch. Many of these foods overlap with the other healthy choices you're making (fiber, healthy fats), so you get a synergistic benefit. If needed, a magnesium supplement at bedtime can help with relaxation, but focus on food first. Ensuring you have enough magnesium can support nerve function, muscle relaxation, and a stable mood – all elements of a well-functioning parasympathetic (vagal) response.

By integrating these tips into your daily life, you're doing more than just fueling your body – you're engaging the "rest and digest" powers of the vagus nerve at every meal. Over time, these habits can lead to a noticeable improvement in how you feel. Many people report not only better digestion (less bloating, more regularity) but also improvements in sleep and stress resilience once they start living a "vagus-friendly" lifestyle. The beauty of the vagus lifestyle is that it's inherently balanced: it's not an extreme diet or a punishing regime, but rather a gentle, enjoyable approach to taking care of yourself. You'll find that when your gut is happy, your mind often follows – perhaps you'll have more energy in the mornings, or a lighter mood throughout the day. This is the natural healing power we all have within us: by making daily choices that promote vagal tone, we give our body permission to heal, recover, and thrive.

As you continue your journey through *The Vagus Lifestyle*, remember that small daily actions lead to big changes in vagal tone and well-being. Every deep breath before a meal, every forkful of fiber-rich veggies, every night of good sleep – they all add up. The gut-brain axis is always listening and responding. By nourishing it with calm and care, you're essentially tuning a magnificent instrument – your nervous system – to play in harmony with your life. In the next chapters, we'll explore even more ways to enrich this mind-body connection. For now, take heart (and stomach): *your vagus nerve has your back*, and with a few simple habits, you can keep this life-giving nerve strong and singing for years to come.

# Chapter 7

# The Vagus Lifestyle in Action – Your Daily Plan for Long-Term Wellness

## Designing Your Day for Vagal Health

Imagine waking up to a day intentionally designed to keep your vagus nerve engaged from dawn to dusk. The "vagus lifestyle" is all about weaving simple, healthful habits into your routine. Let's walk through a sample day optimized for vagal tone, showing how ordinary activities – morning breathing, afternoon movement, and evening relaxation – become opportunities for better health.

**Morning:** Start your day by gently stimulating your vagus nerve with a few minutes of deep breathing or meditation. Before reaching for your phone or diving into emails, sit comfortably and take 5 minutes for diaphragmatic breathing. Inhale slowly through your nose, feeling your belly rise, then exhale even more slowly through your mouth. This simple practice activates the vagus nerve and shifts your body into "rest and digest" mode. Research shows that even a few minutes of deep, belly breathing can lower stress hormones and heart rate, priming you for a calmer day. You might try a breathing technique like *4-7-8 breathing* (inhale for 4 counts, hold for 7, exhale for 8) or Cedars-Sinai's tip of inhaling for six counts and exhaling for eight. Such exercises stimulate vagal activity and have an almost immediate relaxing effect – reducing anxiety and blood pressure while boosting mental clarity. If you enjoy meditation, these same morning minutes can be spent quietly observing your breath or practicing mindfulness. Meditation not only activates the vagus nerve but also calms the networks that drive our stress response. As one neurologist notes, meditation can lower heart rate and blood pressure, engaging the vagus to unlock a *relaxation response*. By starting the morning with intentional calm, you're essentially "tuning" your nervous system for resilience, so minor stresses later on won't throw you off balance.

**Midday:** Throughout the day, look for small chances to reset and recharge your vagal tone. Modern life often keeps us in sympathetic "fight or flight" overdrive through constant emails, meetings, and to-do lists. Counteract this by sprinkling mini vagus-friendly breaks into your schedule. For example, mid-morning or lunchtime, take a 5-minute breathing break – push your chair back, close your eyes, and take a dozen slow, mindful breaths. These short pauses shift your focus from mental chatter to bodily rhythm, activating the vagus and dissolving tension. You could also try a quick self-massage or gentle stretch at your desk. A brief neck and shoulder massage stimulates vagal pathways and can lower a pounding heart rate or racing thoughts almost on the spot. If you have the flexibility, step outside for a few minutes of fresh air and natural light. A short walk around the block, especially in a green environment, is doubly beneficial: mild aerobic exercise plus the calming influence of nature. Mild physical activity and even a simple nature walk engage the parasympathetic system, helping your body regulate stress and return to baseline. Think of these little habits as "vagal snacks" – small, frequent nourishment for your nervous system that keep you centered and energized through the busiest of days.

**Afternoon:** At some point, aim for a longer bout of movement – ideally an exercise session that you enjoy. Endurance activities like jogging, cycling, swimming, or a brisk 30-minute walk are perfect for stimulating vagus nerve activity and lifting your mood. In fact, Cedars-Sinai experts note that aerobic exercise is a powerful vagal toning tool: research suggests endurance and interval training significantly boost vagus nerve signals and parasympathetic control in the brain. This may explain the "runner's high" that athletes report during long runs – that blissful feeling is partly the vagus nerve at work! You don't have to be a marathoner to reap the benefits, though. Simply getting your heart rate up with moderate exercise sends signals through the vagus that help regulate heart rhythm, improve circulation, and release mood-enhancing neurotransmitters. One clinical supervisor explains that *"exercise stimulates the vagus nerve with hormonal responses, which lead to benefits for the brain and mental health."* When you work out, your body pumps out endorphins, serotonin and dopamine – chemicals that reduce stress and create feelings of happiness. Pair that neurochemical boost with vagal activation, and you have a recipe for lower anxiety and a brighter mood. For example, you might schedule a jog or bike ride in the late afternoon to shake off work stress. If high-intensity workouts aren't your style, even a light cycling session or dancing to music in your living room counts – any movement that gently elevates your heart rate improves vagal tone. The key is consistency. Experts recommend accumulating about 150 minutes a week of moderate exercise (such as 30 minutes, 5 days a week) to keep your vagus nerve—and heart—robust. This could be a brisk walk during your lunch break or a casual bike ride after work. Over time, these active afternoons will pay off: higher vagal tone, better cardiovascular health, and a noticeably sunnier outlook on life.

*Afternoon exercise, like a friendly jog or bike ride, not only elevates your mood but also stimulates vagus nerve activity. Aerobic activities send calming parasympathetic signals through your body, which can reduce stress and even give you that "runner's high" glow.*

**Evening:** As the day winds down, your vagus nerve becomes an ally in transitioning into restful sleep. In the evening, try to unplug from screens and engage in screen-free relaxation at least an hour before bed. This is important because the blue light and mental stimulation from devices can keep your sympathetic nervous system wired, making it harder for the vagus nerve to do its calming work. Instead, consider creating a soothing pre-bed routine that signals safety and relaxation to your body. Dimming the lights, playing soft music, or practicing gentle yoga stretches are all excellent ways to activate the vagus nerve at day's end. Gentle stretching, for instance, releases tension from your muscles and can stimulate vagal pathways that help slow your heart rate and breathing. You might spend 10 minutes doing slow neck rolls, spinal twists, or legs-up-the-wall pose – all while breathing deeply. Some people also find humming or singing to be surprisingly relaxing at night; the vibrations from vocalizing can engage the vagus nerve through connections in the throat, signaling the brain that it's okay to unwind. Another wonderfully calming habit is taking a warm bath in the evening.

Immersing yourself in warm water coaxes your nervous system into a parasympathetic state – your muscles relax, blood vessels dilate, and your heart rate naturally slows as warmth envelops you. This heat-induced relaxation activates vagal tone in a gentle way, similar to how a sauna does, but in the comfort of your tub. One wellness coach notes that using a sauna or warm bath at home is a great method to "relax your muscles and activate parasympathetic relaxation," yielding vagal benefits without the shock of cold exposure. Try adding Epsom salts or a few drops of lavender oil to your bath for extra calming effect; as you soak for 15–20 minutes, practice slow breathing to double up the vagus stimulation. By the time you towel off, you'll likely feel your body shifted into a quiet, safe mode ready for sleep. Finally, when you get into bed, you can even do a final breathing exercise (like a few rounds of 4-7-8 breathing or simple belly breathing) to signal to your vagus nerve – and your racing mind – that it's truly time to rest. With these habits, your evening routine becomes a ritual of vagal activation, helping you fall asleep faster and sleep more deeply. Indeed, activating the vagus nerve at night can lower cortisol and improve overall sleep quality. As you dim the lights and let go of the day's worries, you're essentially inviting your vagus nerve to guide you into a peaceful, restorative night.

By mapping these practices onto a typical day, you can see how easily the vagus lifestyle fits in. Your morning breathwork, daytime movement, and evening wind-down aren't "extra" tasks – they fold naturally into daily routines, turning ordinary moments into healing opportunities. Over time, this structured daily routine will feel almost second-nature. Each day becomes a balanced cycle: you energize and de-stress in turn, all the while strengthening your body's natural relaxation response. The cumulative effect is profound. Instead of running on stress and adrenaline, you're training your nervous system to operate in a state of balance. Little by little, these vagal-friendly habits build resilience. And as you'll see next, real people have transformed their health by consistently living this "vagus lifestyle."

## Lessons from Success Stories

Throughout this book we've followed the journeys of several individuals – people from different walks of life who all had one thing in common: they needed a change to reclaim their health. By embracing daily vagus-friendly habits, each of them experienced tangible, life-changing improvements. Let's revisit a few of these inspiring stories (with names changed for privacy) and see how far they've come. Their successes are living proof that these simple practices, done consistently, can yield dramatic results, whether you're a total beginner or a seasoned wellness enthusiast.

**Reducing Blood Pressure and Anxiety:** One success story is a 45-year-old executive who we'll call *"M."* M had struggled with hypertension and chronic anxiety for years, a byproduct of her high-stress job. In Chapter 3, we learned how stress overdrive and poor vagal tone were keeping her blood pressure elevated and her nerves on edge. M decided to implement two core vagus lifestyle habits: daily breathing exercises and evening yoga. Every morning before work, she practiced 10 minutes of deep breathing (focusing on slow exhales), and each evening she did a 20-minute gentle yoga routine to unwind. The first couple of weeks were challenging – breaking the habit of reaching for her phone in the morning or TV at night – but she persisted. After a few months, the changes were remarkable. M's blood pressure, which used to hover in the borderline high range, dropped significantly into the normal range, surprising even her doctor. It wasn't magic; it was physiology. Slow, deep breathing and yoga both activate the vagus nerve, which in turn helps dilate blood vessels and reduce blood pressure. In fact, clinical research backs this up: yoga interventions of a few months can produce measurable reductions in blood pressure for patients with hypertension. M's anxiety levels also plummeted. She reported that she no longer felt "on edge" all the time – those daily breathing breaks taught her body how to release tension and engage the calm response on cue. Biologically, what likely happened is that her consistent practice raised her vagal tone (as evidenced by a lower resting heart rate and higher heart rate variability), making her less reactive to stress triggers. As one therapist explained, *"Deep and slow breathing activates the vagus nerves and leads to a reduction in anxiety and stress responses."* M's calmer mind and improved cardiovascular stats illustrate just how powerful these habits can be. Importantly, these changes weren't achieved through medication or major lifestyle overhauls – they came from harnessing the body's natural relaxation circuitry. M's story shows that even if you're juggling a busy career, finding a few minutes for your vagus nerve each day can shift your entire baseline of health.

**Easing Autoimmune Symptoms with Mind-Body Medicine:** Another compelling story from earlier chapters was that of *"J.,"* a 34-year-old dealing with an autoimmune condition. J suffered from an autoimmune thyroid disorder that left her fatigued, inflamed, and often in pain. Traditional medical treatment helped some, but she was still struggling with flare-ups and stress, which tended to exacerbate her symptoms. In Chapter 5, we followed J's decision to complement her medical therapy with mind-body practices aimed at nurturing her vagus nerve. She started with simple meditation for 15 minutes a day, and later added tai chi classes twice a week to introduce gentle movement and breathing into her routine. The rationale was clear: practices like meditation and tai chi can engage the vagus nerve, thereby reducing the chronic "fight or flight" activation that worsens inflammation. At first, J wondered if such subtle habits could really influence something as formidable as an autoimmune disease. But by the time we talked to her again for this chapter, she was a believer. After four months of consistent practice, J noticed a significant decrease in the frequency and intensity of her flare-ups. Her digestion improved and she had more energy. Even her inflammatory markers (like C-reactive protein) trended down on her lab tests. How might this be happening? Science offers some clues. The vagus nerve is a key regulator of the immune system and inflammation – it helps prevent the release of excessive pro-inflammatory cytokines that drive autoimmune flares. When J activated her vagus nerve through daily meditation and the flowing movements of tai chi, she was essentially tapping into an "anti-inflammatory reflex" in her body. In fact, researchers have found that enhancing vagal tone can reduce chronic inflammation and support the body's healing in conditions ranging from rheumatoid arthritis to irritable bowel syndrome. J herself describes it in simpler terms: "When I'm meditating, I can feel my body relaxing and my stomach unclenching. It's like I'm telling my immune system,

'Everything's okay.'" Over time, that message seems to have gotten through – her immune system is quieter, and she feels more in control of her condition. J's journey illustrates that combining conventional medicine with vagus-friendly lifestyle changes can create a powerful synergy. By using meditation as "medicine," she not only improved her symptoms but also gained a coping tool that she can carry for life. It reinforces a hopeful message: even with an autoimmune illness, you are not powerless. By engaging the mind-body connection and vagus nerve, you can influence your immune system and reclaim a measure of control over your health destiny.

**Conquering Lifelong Insomnia:** For years, *"S."* thought he was just a "bad sleeper." This fifty-something reader from Chapter 6 had battled chronic insomnia – taking hours to fall asleep and waking up multiple times a night. He had tried various remedies with limited success, until he learned about the vagus nerve's role in sleep regulation. S decided to overhaul his nighttime routine into a vagus-centric ritual. He set a consistent bedtime and, for an hour before, committed to screen-free, relaxing activities. He would dim the lights, do some light stretches and breathing exercises, and sometimes listen to calming music. Additionally, S experimented with brief cold exposure (a vagus nerve hack he'd read about): each night he splashed his face and neck with cold water, stimulating the "diving reflex" known to activate the vagus and slow the heart rate for sleep. The changes were gradual, but by the third or fourth week, S reported an astounding development – he was regularly sleeping through the night. Falling asleep became easier (sometimes just 15 minutes instead of over an hour), and he woke up feeling rested for the first time in decades. His secret? Teaching his body to consistently activate the parasympathetic, sleep-friendly state at night. Turning off screens and doing breathing exercises helped trigger the vagal response that makes you drowsy (lowering heart rate and cortisol), rather than the stress response that would have kept him tossing and turning. Even the quick cold splash contributed: exposure to cold can increase vagus nerve activity and has been shown to redirect blood flow and slow pulse, preparing the body for rest. One sleep specialist we cited explained that vagus nerve stimulation "shifts the body into a restful state" by tapping into the parasympathetic system, which is exactly what S experienced. His case demonstrates how good sleep hygiene paired with vagal techniques can break the cycle of insomnia. By respecting the body's natural rhythms and helping them along (through vagus activation), S essentially retrained his nervous system to downshift at night. Now he guards his evening routine religiously, saying it's become a cherished wind-down time. No longer does he label himself a "bad sleeper" – he's empowered by the knowledge that he can control his own physiology to get the rest he needs.

Each of these success stories – lower blood pressure, calmer autoimmunity, and sweeter sleep – highlights a different benefit of the vagus lifestyle. Yet they all share a common thread: consistent, daily habits were the catalyst for change. These individuals did not see overnight miracles; rather, they saw steady progress that snowballed into dramatic improvement over months. Their journeys show that *anyone* can benefit from vagal tuning, whether you're addressing a serious health issue or just seeking better wellness. Importantly, the vagus lifestyle meets you where you are. If you're a beginner, you can start with one small habit (like M's morning breathing practice) and still see results. If you're already health-conscious, you can layer these practices on top of your existing routine to reach new heights of well-being. The take-home lesson is clear: our bodies want to heal and find balance, and by engaging the vagus nerve we give them the nudge they need to do so. These real-world outcomes are motivating – they remind us that we're not at the mercy of stress or illness. By making conscious daily choices, we truly can rewrite our health story, just like M, J, and S did.

## Expert Roundup – Top Tips for Longevity

As we near the end of our journey, let's bolster our motivation with some parting advice from experts across different fields. Think of this as a quick roundup of top tips for long-term health and longevity, all seen through the lens of caring for your vagus nerve. We've gathered wisdom from a cardiologist, a psychologist, and a sleep researcher – three authoritative voices echoing the core guidance of this book. Their perspectives reinforce why maintaining good vagal tone is so vital and offer memorable takeaways to carry forward.

**Heart Health and Longevity – The Cardiologist's Tip:** From a cardiology standpoint, one of the best indicators of longevity is your heart rate variability (HRV) – essentially a measure of vagal tone and how balanced your autonomic nervous system is. A cardiologist might remind us that maintaining a high vagal tone (and thus high HRV) is linked to better cardiovascular health and a longer life. In simple terms, when your vagus nerve is strong, your heart beats more flexibly (adjusting to stresses and relaxation appropriately), which is protective for your heart over the long run. Research backs this up: studies have found that people with *lower* resting heart rates and *greater* heart rate variability tend to experience fewer cardiac events and may even live longer lives. Conversely, decreased HRV (a sign of poor vagal function) correlates with higher risks of hypertension, heart disease, and even increased mortality. In fact, clinicians at the Hospital for Special Surgery note that a well-functioning parasympathetic system can reduce your risk of heart disease and stroke and possibly even extend your lifespan. So, the expert's advice is clear: exercise regularly, practice stress reduction, and take care of your vagus nerve as part of your heart-health regimen. By aiming for that balanced "rest and digest" state more often, you're not just feeling calmer – you're literally helping your heart last longer. Next time you finish a breathing session or yoga class, consider that you've given your heart a dose of longevity medicine. As one cardiologist put it, *a strong vagal tone is like a secret weapon for healthy aging*, keeping your heart young and resilient well into your golden years.

**Mood and Social Connection – The Psychologist's Tip:** Mental health professionals have long recognized the interplay between the vagus nerve and our emotional well-being. A psychologist's top tip might surprise you in its simplicity: laugh often and nurture your social bonds. Why? Because social connection and genuine laughter are powerful activators of the vagus nerve, and they come with a cascade of positive effects. When you engage in heartfelt social interaction – whether it's a deep conversation with a friend or a big belly laugh at a silly joke – you are sending your body signals of safety and happiness, which the vagus nerve translates into a calming parasympathetic response. Laughter, in particular, has been called "internal jogging." A good, hearty laugh massages your internal organs, slows your breathing (as you exhale those "ha ha's"), and stimulates the vagal fibers in your diaphragm and throat. This is why after a bout of laughter, you often feel relaxed and content. One expert noted that even *watching a 5-minute comedy video that makes you laugh can reinforce the parasympathetic system*, immediately shifting you into a state of positive relaxation. Social bonding has a similar effect: hugging a loved one, for example, can boost vagal activity by releasing oxytocin (the bonding hormone) and lowering stress hormones. In essence, love and laughter are medicine for the vagus nerve. A clinical therapist might advise: make time each week to connect with people who uplift you – have a phone call that makes you smile or a game night with friends. And don't underestimate laughter as a therapeutic tool. As the University of Virginia's health blog quipped, if you want to stimulate your vagus nerve, aim for those deep belly laughs – *"It really is good medicine"*. The psychological benefit is two-fold: you increase vagal tone in the moment, and you also buffer yourself against future stress by fostering a sense of social safety and support. Remember, the vagus nerve is intricately tied into our social engagement system (it's even part of why heart rate calms when we feel socially supported). So by following this expert tip – prioritizing connection and humor – you nourish your nervous system in a delightfully enjoyable way.

**Rest and Recovery – The Sleep Researcher's Tip:** Finally, let's hear from the perspective of a sleep expert, who would emphasize the foundational role of consistent, quality sleep in vagal health (and vice versa). A sleep researcher's advice might be: *keep a regular sleep schedule and develop a calming bedtime routine to support your vagus nerve and overall wellness.* We've learned that during deep sleep, the parasympathetic system (via the vagus nerve) dominates – your heart rate slows, blood pressure drops, and the body enters a profound state of restoration. This is when healing and memory consolidation occur. But to reap those benefits, you need to allow your body to get *into* that parasympathetic state each night. That's where good sleep habits come in. Experts recommend aiming for 7–9 hours of sleep per night and keeping your bedtime and wake-up time consistent, even on weekends. This consistency trains your circadian rhythm and makes it easier for your vagus nerve to guide you into sleep. The researcher would also stress creating a calming pre-sleep routine: perhaps dim the lights, do some light reading or listen to soothing music, and crucially, minimize screen time before bed. The reason is twofold – screens emit blue light that can disrupt your melatonin (sleep hormone) production, and absorbing work emails or news at 10 pm can spike your stress, counteracting vagal activation. By contrast, a tech-free wind-down (think of a warm shower, gentle stretching, or journaling) can signal your vagus nerve that it's safe to power the system down. One wellness resource encapsulated this advice well: *"Aim for 7–9 hours of sleep per night. Create a calming bedtime routine, keep a consistent sleep schedule, and minimize screen time before bed."* These steps help ensure that when you do fall asleep, you slip quickly into that parasympathetic-dominant, healing sleep. The payoff? Not only will you feel more refreshed, but you'll also be supporting your vagal tone. Poor or irregular sleep can lower vagal activity and raise stress levels, whereas consistent quality sleep boosts vagal function, creating a virtuous cycle of better rest and better resilience. In short, the sleep expert's longevity tip is: protect your sleep like the precious medicine it is. By doing so, you give your vagus nerve nightly tune-ups, which in turn will help you stay healthier and more energetic during your days.

These expert tips, taken together, provide a well-rounded capstone for the vagus lifestyle. A cardiologist urges balancing the nervous system for a long life, a psychologist encourages joyful connections for mental well-being, and a sleep researcher reminds us that recovery is just as important as activity. Although they approach it from different angles, the underlying theme is unified: nurturing your vagus nerve leads to a longer, healthier, and happier life. High vagal tone is like the thread stitching together heart health, emotional health, and restorative sleep. By remembering these simple yet profound tips – keep your heart rate variability up, laugh and love more, and honor your sleep – you carry forward the wisdom of this book, reinforced by experts, as you continue your wellness journey.

## Putting It All Together – Your Roadmap to Wellness

Now that you've learned the science and the practices, it's time to put it all together into an actionable plan. Think of this final section as your roadmap to long-term wellness. Adopting a new lifestyle is always a challenge, but breaking it down into manageable steps can make the process enjoyable and sustainable. Here, we present a simple four-week challenge to kick-start your "vagus lifestyle," along with a checklist of core habits to maintain moving forward. By the end of these four weeks, you'll have integrated breathing, movement, relaxation, and other key elements into your daily life – setting you up for lasting health benefits. Remember, consistency is more important than perfection. Even small, proactive steps can yield profound improvements in well-being. Let's chart your course:

- **Week 1: Breathe and Reset:** In the first week, focus on building awareness of your breath and incorporating daily breathing exercises. Each morning (or evening, if that suits you better), spend 5–10 minutes on deep breathing practice. Use the techniques you learned – for example, 4-7-8 breathing or simply slow diaphragmatic breaths where your exhale is longer than your inhale. Your goal this week is to do this every day, even if some days it's only a few minutes. Additionally, start noticing your breath during the day. Whenever you catch yourself stressed (tight chest, shallow breaths), take a short breathing break: inhale deeply and exhale slowly, for just 3 or 4 cycles. By week's end, you should notice you're more tuned in to your body's signals. You might even feel a bit calmer overall as your nervous system begins to adapt to these mini "resets." Jot down a few notes each day about your mood and energy after breathing; it will motivate you as you see patterns. *Habit checklist:* Daily morning breathing exercise; one mini breathing break during work hours; try one session of humming or chanting on a day you feel anxious (just to see how it affects you).

- **Week 2: Add Daily Movement:** In the second week, continue your breathing practice and add daily walks or other light exercise to your routine. The aim is at least 20–30 minutes of physical activity that mildly elevates your heart rate. Choose activities you enjoy – maybe a brisk walk in a park, a leisurely bike ride, or a beginner yoga flow. If you already work out regularly, great; focus on the *quality* of your movement, keeping it mindful and noting afterward how relaxed or uplifted you feel. If you're new to exercise, start small: even a 15-minute walk around your neighborhood after lunch or dinner is excellent. This week is about finding joy in movement and realizing it's not a chore but a natural way to stimulate your vagus nerve and boost your mood. Invite a friend or family member to join you if possible, combining exercise with social connection (two vagus boosters in one!). By the end of Week 2, you might notice improvements like better focus during the day or more stable energy. That's the magic of moving your body – you're pumping oxygen and endorphins, while also strengthening that calming parasympathetic tone. *Habit checklist:* Continue daily breathing exercises; 20–30 minutes of moderate activity each day (walking counts!); take one "nature walk" this week if you can, immersing yourself in a green environment for vagus benefits; end a couple of workouts with 5 minutes of gentle stretching and deep breaths as a cooldown to really tap into the vagus.

- **Week 3: Refine Your Evening Routine:** In the third week, keep up the breathing and exercise, and now turn your attention to improving your evening and sleep routine. Good sleep is crucial, and this week you'll create habits that optimize your vagus activation at night. Start by setting a consistent bedtime and sticking to it (even on weekends, aim not to stray by more than ~30 minutes). Next, establish a screen-free wind-down period before bed – begin with 30 minutes and try to extend it to an hour by week's end. Use that time for relaxing activities: light stretches, a warm bath, reading a physical book, journaling, or meditation. Consider incorporating one of the vagal stimulators we discussed: maybe try a warm bath one evening with Epsom salts (to relax muscles and calm the nervous system), and on another night do a session of progressive muscle relaxation or guided meditation. Also, pay attention to your bedroom environment – make it cool, dark, and peaceful, which helps signal safety to your brain for sleep. If racing thoughts are an issue at night, remember to use breathing techniques then, too. By the end of Week 3, you should notice you're falling asleep faster or sleeping more soundly. Some people report dramatically fewer middle-of-the-night awakenings just from cutting out late-night screen time (blue light and stimulation were sabotaging their vagal tone before bed). Continue to note changes in a journal: Are you feeling sleepier at bedtime? More refreshed in the morning? This feedback will reinforce why these habits matter. *Habit checklist:* Maintain Weeks 1–2 practices; set a regular bedtime/wake time; institute a 30–60 minute pre-bed relaxation routine (no screens); include at least one of the following each night – breathing exercise, gentle stretching, or a warm bath; if you struggle with insomnia one night, try the cold water splash trick or legs-up-the-wall pose and see if it helps calm you.

- **Week 4: Integrate Diet and Social Well-Being:** In the final week of the challenge, you'll round out your vagus lifestyle by looking at diet and social connections – two areas that also influence vagal tone. First, diet: this week, aim to make some pro-inflammatory to anti-inflammatory swaps in your meals. For instance, try to incorporate foods rich in omega-3 fatty acids (like salmon, chia seeds or walnuts) as they can support heart and nerve health. Pile your plate with fiber-rich vegetables and fermented foods (yogurt, kefir, sauerkraut) which promote a healthy gut microbiome – remember, the vagus nerve connects to our gut and a healthy gut can improve vagal signaling. At the same time, reduce stimulants and processed foods: too much caffeine, sugar, or heavy refined meals can keep your system in high alert. Instead, favor balanced meals with protein, healthy fats, and complex carbs to keep blood sugar steady and stress low. The idea isn't a strict diet but rather nourishing your body in a way that complements your mind-body work. Second, focus on social and emotional well-being. Set a goal to engage in at least one uplifting social interaction each day – this could be calling a friend, playing with your pet, or having lunch with a coworker. Notice how positive social contact makes you feel safe and happy; that's the vagus nerve at play. Also, laugh out loud this week! Watch a comedy special or recall some funny memories.

Laughter truly is a vagus tonic, as experts shared, increasing heart rate variability and easing stress. If you haven't already, Week 4 is also a great time to experiment with any vagal techniques you're curious about: maybe you try a morning cold shower once or twice, or you attend that community yoga class or singing group. These experiences can keep things fresh and reveal additional tools you enjoy. By the end of this week, step back and applaud yourself – you've practiced four weeks of the vagus lifestyle! Most importantly, you've personalized it. You've discovered which breathing exercises calm you best, which exercise you actually look forward to, and how much better you feel when you stick to a healthy sleep pattern and diet. *Habit checklist:* Continue Weeks 1–3 habits (they should be feeling pretty ingrained by now); incorporate gut-friendly, whole foods into each day; limit junk food and stimulants (perhaps no coffee after noon, as a test); schedule social time or phone calls with loved ones; do something that makes you laugh every day (yes, memes count); try any "bonus" vagus technique that intrigues you (humming in the shower, foot reflexology massage, etc.).

By the end of this 4-week challenge, you will have a solid foundation. Of course, life will continue beyond these weeks, and the idea is not to be perfect every day but to have a toolkit of healthy habits you can rely on. As you move forward, you can mix and match these practices as needed. Some days might be heavy on stress – that's when you know to lean on extra breathing exercises and maybe a cold splash for a quick reset. Other days you'll feel great and can pay it forward by, say, engaging in more social connection or exploring advanced practices like meditation retreats or biofeedback for HRV. Your vagus nerve will continue to strengthen with use, much like a muscle. In fact, you might find that what used to throw you into anxiety or fatigue no longer has the same effect – that's a sign your baseline vagal tone has improved, granting you a buffer against stress.

As we conclude, let's reiterate the core promise that has been unfolding throughout this book: by understanding and consistently nurturing your vagus nerve, you have gained a powerful tool to control your health destiny. You've learned that the vagus nerve is not just another nerve in the body; it's a master regulator linking your brain with your heart, lungs, gut, and more. And critically, it's a part of your physiology that you can influence through conscious habits. This is incredibly empowering. It means that to a large extent, longevity, good sleep, and healing are not out of your hands – they respond to the lifestyle you live. By adopting the vagus lifestyle, you are stacking the odds in your favor for a longer and more vibrant life. Even medical institutions note how enhanced vagal tone is associated with lower risk of major killers like heart disease and with greater resilience against illness. You are actively working to help yourself *live longer, sleep more peacefully,* and *unlock your body's natural healing power* through these daily choices. For instance, maintaining strong vagal activity can help keep your blood pressure and inflammation levels low, contributing to a healthier, potentially longer life. Activating the vagus nerve regularly leads to better sleep quality and mood stability. And by modulating inflammation via the vagus, you support your body's innate ability to recover and heal. All these translate to years added to life and life added to years.

In closing, remember that wellness is a journey, not a destination. There will be days you falter or feel unmotivated – that's okay. Use those moments as reminders of why you started. Perhaps reread the success stories for inspiration or recall an expert's words that resonated with you. Know that even small steps make a difference. One expert from Mass General beautifully noted that taking even 5–10 minutes a day for practices that calm your senses can make a *huge* difference in your stress levels and health. It's true. Consistency, not intensity, is what yields lasting change. You now have an array of small, simple habits – your breathing, your walks, your laughter, your evening wind-down – which, when practiced regularly, will compound into profound benefits. Trust the process and trust your body's wisdom. Over time, you'll likely notice not just physical improvements (like fewer headaches or better digestion or deeper sleep) but also a shift in how you approach life – perhaps with more patience, optimism, and gratitude. This is the transformative power of the vagus lifestyle.

Congratulations on equipping yourself with this knowledge and for taking charge of your well-being. The vagus nerve may be the "wandering nerve," but you now have it firmly on your side as a guide toward wellness. As you continue on your path, keep listening to your body's signals and keep practicing the habits that make you feel balanced and strong. In doing so, you are actively shaping a healthier, happier future for yourself. Here's to living longer, sleeping better, and thriving with the power of the vagus lifestyle in action – for years to come!

# Epilogue

Your vagus nerve has been waiting patiently for this moment—the moment when you finally understand that healing happens not through dramatic interventions, but through the gentle, consistent practices you now hold in your hands.

As you close this book, you carry with you more than information. You possess a roadmap to your body's most sophisticated healing system, one that has evolved over millions of years to restore, repair, and renew. Every deep breath you take, every moment of gratitude you cultivate, every cold shower you embrace, sends signals along this remarkable neural highway, telling your body that safety and healing are possible.

The practices outlined in these pages—from vagal breathing and meditation to mindful movement and restorative sleep—represent humanity's rediscovery of ancient wisdom through modern science. Your ancestors knew instinctively what researchers now measure in laboratories: that true health emerges when we create the conditions for our parasympathetic nervous system to flourish.

Some days, the practices will feel effortless. Others, they may seem like small acts of rebellion against a culture that prizes stress over serenity. Remember that each conscious choice to activate your vagus nerve creates ripples of healing that extend far beyond yourself, touching your relationships, your community, and even future generations through epigenetic changes.

The vagus lifestyle begins with a single breath, a moment of stillness, a choice to prioritize your body's innate wisdom over external demands. As you embark on this journey, trust that your nervous system is already responding, already healing, already guiding you toward the vibrant health that is your birthright.

Your transformation starts now. Your vagus nerve is ready. The question that remains is beautifully simple: are you?

www.ingramcontent.com/pod-product-compliance
Lightning Source LLC
Chambersburg PA
CBHW070121030426
42335CB00016B/2230